Doctors Lim and Burton offer a concise and easy-to-read review of the latest research regarding the prevention and treatment of pediatric obesity. This book offers critical guidance, given that pediatric obesity is a widespread public health concern with long-term mental and physical health consequences. An interprofessional approach to prevention strategies and lifestyle interventions, this book is a necessary read for a wide range of health care professionals.

—**Wendy L. Ward, PhD, ABPP, FAPA, FNAP,** Associate Provost for Faculty and Professor in Pediatrics, University of Arkansas for Medical Sciences, Fayetteville, AR; CEO, Ward Coaching and Consulting, LLC

T0367137

Psychological Approaches to the Treatment of Pediatric Obesity

Psychological Approaches to the Treatment of Pediatric Obesity

Crystal S. Lim and
E. Thomaseo Burton

 AMERICAN PSYCHOLOGICAL ASSOCIATION

Published by
American Psychological Association
750 First Street, NE
Washington, DC 20002
https://www.apa.org

Order Department
https://www.apa.org/pubs/books
order@apa.org

Typeset in Charter and Interstate by Circle Graphics, Inc., Reisterstown, MD

Printer: Sheridan Books, Chelsea, MI
Cover Designer: Gwen J. Grafft, Minneapolis, MN

Library of Congress Cataloging-in-Publication Data

Names: Lim, Crystal S., author. | Burton, E. Thomaseo, author.
Title: Psychological approaches to the treatment of pediatric obesity /
   authored by Crystal S. Lim and E. Thomaseo Burton.
Description: Washington, DC : American Psychological Association, [2024] |
   Includes bibliographical references and index.
Identifiers: LCCN 2023044310 (print) | LCCN 2023044311 (ebook) |
   ISBN 9781433838927 (paperback) | ISBN 9781433839184 (ebook)
Subjects: LCSH: Obesity in children--Psychological aspects. | Obesity in
   children--Treatment. | Overweight children--Mental health. | Overweight
   children--Psychology. | BISAC: PSYCHOLOGY / Psychopathology / General |
   MEDICAL / Pediatrics
Classification: LCC RJ399.C6 L56 2024 (print) | LCC RJ399.C6 (ebook) |
   DDC 618.92/398--dc23/eng/20240126
LC record available at https://lccn.loc.gov/2023044310
LC ebook record available at https://lccn.loc.gov/2023044311

https://doi.org/10.1037/0000401-000

Printed in the United States of America

10 9 8 7 6 5 4 3 2 1

Contents

Acknowledgments

We would like to express our most sincere appreciation to the patients and their families with whom we have worked over the years. Thank you for allowing us to be part of your health journeys. You have taught us so much about the complexity and rewards of our work, as well as the importance of humility and persistence. We also would like to thank our own families, friends, and colleagues for their support and encouragement throughout our training and professional pursuits.

Psychological Approaches to the Treatment of Pediatric Obesity

PART I INTRODUCTION TO PEDIATRIC OBESITY

The introductory chapters of this book provide an overview of pediatric obesity and establish the condition as an important public health issue. We present key definitions of pediatric obesity and discuss issues of diversity, health equity, weight stigma, and weight-based discrimination. Finally, we review factors that contribute to onset and maintenance of pediatric obesity, as well as highlight etiological elements that may serve as targets of medical and psychological treatment of the disease.

1 OVERVIEW OF PEDIATRIC OBESITY

Psychological, Public Health, and Diversity Implications

Pediatric obesity is a significant public health concern that is multifaceted in regard to its development, maintenance, and treatment. The purpose of this book is to review psychological factors important to consider in the treatment of pediatric obesity through a health equity and diversity-inclusive lens. The goals of the book are to review treatment strategies, including prevention, lifestyle interventions, medications, and weight loss surgery, specific to pediatric obesity, as well as psychological factors that affect patient and family engagement in prevention and treatment approaches. We also highlight evidence-based treatments for clinical child and adolescent psychology that can be implemented in the treatment of pediatric obesity, as well as review other special considerations, such as body image concerns. The intended audience consists of psychologists, behavioral health practitioners, and trainees who provide care to children and adolescents across various settings (e.g., primary care, mental health clinics, specialty medical settings, schools, community organizations) and who focus on preventing and treating pediatric obesity. Thus, we anticipate readers will have foundational knowledge of and experience with both child clinical psychology and pediatric obesity.

https://doi.org/10.1037/0000401-001
Psychological Approaches to the Treatment of Pediatric Obesity, by C. S. Lim and E. T. Burton

The purpose of this initial chapter is to discuss the format and structure of the book and provide background with regard to defining pediatric obesity and introducing pediatric obesity as a critical public health issue.

The book consists of three main parts: Part I, including this chapter, provides an overview of pediatric obesity, specifically focusing on definitions and evidence of public health impacts, diversity and healthy equity issues, weight stigma and discrimination, and potential causes of obesity development and maintenance that influence medical and psychological treatment of the disease. The chapters in Part II review prevention and treatment approaches to address pediatric obesity in various contexts, such as school-based prevention programs; retail and immersion programs, such as summer camps; and medications and surgical treatments that take place in specialized medical contexts. Part III discusses specific psychological factors, such as comorbid psychological disorders, that are important to consider in pediatric obesity prevention and treatment efforts. We include case study descriptions and a focus on evidence-based psychological treatments that can improve health and psychological outcomes for children and families.[1] Each chapter concludes with "Key Points" to highlight main takeaways, as well as a "Thinking Outside the Box" question intended to provoke deeper thought about content presented in the chapter.

DEFINITION OF PEDIATRIC OBESITY

Before we move on to identifying pediatric obesity as a significant public health issue, it is important to define what we will be referring to throughout the book as "pediatric obesity." First, in adults, the diagnosis of overweight and obesity is generally made by calculating the body mass index (BMI), which is based on height (m) and weight (kg) measurements (i.e., BMI = kg/m^2). For adults in the United States, a diagnosis of overweight is considered a BMI ≥25, and a diagnosis of obesity is considered at BMI ≥30. Severe obesity is diagnosed as a BMI ≥40. Because of expected height and weight growth trajectories in children, BMI and BMI percentiles are calculated on the basis of age- and sex-normed growth charts (Hales et al., 2022; Kuczmarski et al., 2000). In youth, overweight is defined as a BMI ≥85th percentile, and obesity is considered a BMI ≥95th percentile. Severe obesity in youth is diagnosed as ≥120% of the 95th percentile on the U.S. Centers for Disease Control and Prevention extended growth charts (Gulati et al., 2012; Hales et al., 2022).

---

[1]All case studies included in this book are fictional composites or have been disguised to protect confidentiality.

In many clinical and research settings, the BMI and BMI percentile are quick, easy, and inexpensive to implement and are recognized as a reliable proxy for body fat percentage and health outcomes (Nuttall, 2015). Thus, BMI-related values are often the indicator of choice for assessing weight status in both children and adults in a variety of clinical and community-based settings. BMI, BMI percentile, or BMI z score are often primary outcomes of interest in randomized controlled trials examining the efficacy and effectiveness of pediatric prevention and weight management treatments. However, it is also important to recognize there has been debate regarding the utility of BMI calculations for persons with diverse body types, such as athletes. In addition, growth charts were initially developed decades ago primarily with White/Caucasian samples. Previous research that has examined the clinical utility of BMI has also been conducted with samples that lack racial/ethnic diversity that is characteristic of the current and projected U.S. population (Rahman & Berenson, 2010). Thus, there are questions regarding the validity of BMI for use in racially and ethnically diverse populations. For example, associations between body fat and BMI have been found to differ by race and ethnicity in children and adolescents (Freedman et al., 2008). Although a full review of this specific issue is beyond the scope of this book (readers are referred to Nuttall [2015] for additional reading on this topic), BMI is a relevant tool and area of inquiry in clinical efforts to prevent and treat pediatric obesity.

PEDIATRIC OBESITY IS A SIGNIFICANT PUBLIC HEALTH ISSUE

In recent decades, there has been increased recognition that obesity is a significant public health problem in the United States and worldwide. This is in part due to increasing prevalence rates in the prior 50 years and the significant impact felt by national and private health care systems. According to the World Health Organization (WHO, 2021), the number of adults with obesity has tripled since 1975, with more than 1.9 billion adults in the world being considered overweight and 650 million considered obese in 2016. In 2018, more than 42% of U.S. adults were considered obese, and 9% were diagnosed with severe obesity (Hales et al., 2020). In children, the prevalence of overweight and obesity has risen tenfold since 1975 (H. J. Lim et al., 2020); specifically, more than 39 million children under age 5 years, and 340 million youth ages 5 to 19 years, were considered overweight or obese in 2016 (WHO, 2021). Figure 1.1 compares surveillance prevalence data of obesity and severe obesity in youth ages 2 to 19 years in the United States from 1999 to 2018 (Ogden et al., 2020).

FIGURE 1.1. Obesity and Severe Obesity Prevalence Rates in U.S. Youth 2 to 19 Years of Age, 1999–2002 to 2015–2018

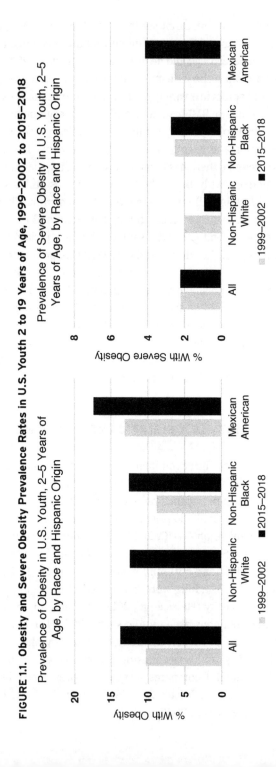

FIGURE 1.1. Obesity and Severe Obesity Prevalence Rates in U.S. Youth 2 to 19 Years of Age, 1999–2002 to 2015–2018 (Continued)

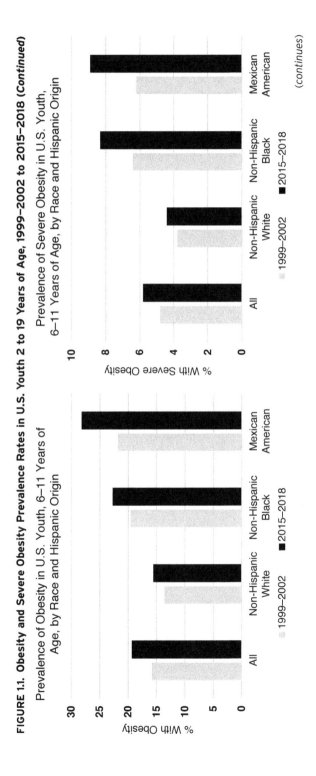

Prevalence of Obesity in U.S. Youth, 6–11 Years of Age, by Race and Hispanic Origin

Prevalence of Severe Obesity in U.S. Youth, 6–11 Years of Age, by Race and Hispanic Origin

(continues)

FIGURE 1.1. Obesity and Severe Obesity Prevalence Rates in U.S. Youth 2 to 19 Years of Age, 1999–2002 to 2015-2018 (*Continued*)

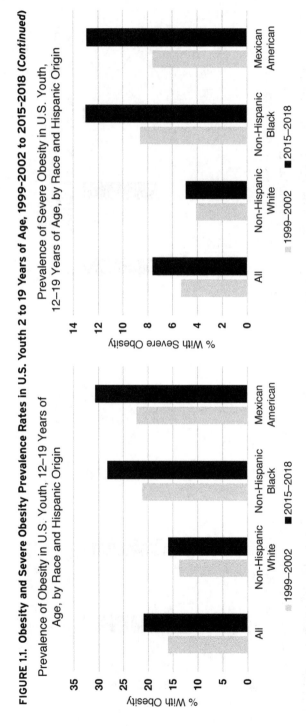

Note. This figure was created on the basis of information presented in Ogden et al. (2020).

In the United States, there are also substantial racial and ethnic differences regarding the prevalence of obesity and severe obesity. For example, Mexican American men and non-Hispanic Black women have the highest rates of obesity, and Mexican American men have experienced a more rapid increase in obesity prevalence compared with non-Hispanic White men (Ogden et al., 2020). In U.S. adolescents, the increased obesity prevalence is largely attributed to prevalence increases in non-Hispanic Black and Mexican American youth (Ogden et al., 2020). We incorporate a health equity and diversity lens throughout this book to help psychologists and other behavioral health practitioners understand the role race/ethnicity and other social determinants of health play in the prevention, development, treatment, and intractability of pediatric obesity.

Overweight and obesity have long-term impacts on morbidity and mortality. Worldwide, more people are affected by obesity than by malnutrition and underweight (WHO, 2021). In addition, obesity is attributed to more than 4 million deaths a year (WHO, 2021). Obesity affects every major organ system in the body, such as cardiovascular (i.e., high blood pressure), metabolic (i.e., dyslipidemia, type 2 diabetes), pulmonary (i.e., asthma, sleep apnea), gastrointestinal (i.e., nonalcoholic fatty liver disease, reflux), skeletal (i.e., Blount disease), and fertility (i.e., polycystic ovary syndrome) problems (Daniels, 2006; see Figure 1.2). In 2008, it was estimated that medical costs associated with obesity in the United States would cost more than $147 billion a year (Finkelstein et al., 2009). Health care costs attributed specifically to pediatric obesity are estimated to be over $14 billion per year (Trasande & Chatterjee, 2009). However, many indirect costs and impacts are not reflected in these estimates.

Research has demonstrated that children with obesity experience significant reductions in health-related quality of life, similar, in fact, to that experienced by children with cancer undergoing chemotherapy (Schwimmer et al., 2003). In addition, overweight and obesity puts children at risk for numerous psychosocial issues, such as bullying, depression, anxiety, behavioral problems, and suicidal ideation (C. S. Lim et al., 2015; Puhl & King, 2013; F. Wang & Veugelers, 2008; Zeller et al., 2006). The American Medical Association officially recognized obesity as a chronic medical condition in 2013, an act that signified decades of work demonstrating the complexity and chronicity of the disease (Kyle et al., 2016). Thus, like other pediatric chronic medical conditions, pediatric obesity requires comprehensive medical and psychological assessments and a chronic course of treatment.

Despite prevention and treatment efforts, prevalence rates of overweight and obesity in adults and youth, as well as health care costs, are expected to

FIGURE 1.2. Physical Health Impacts of Pediatric Obesity

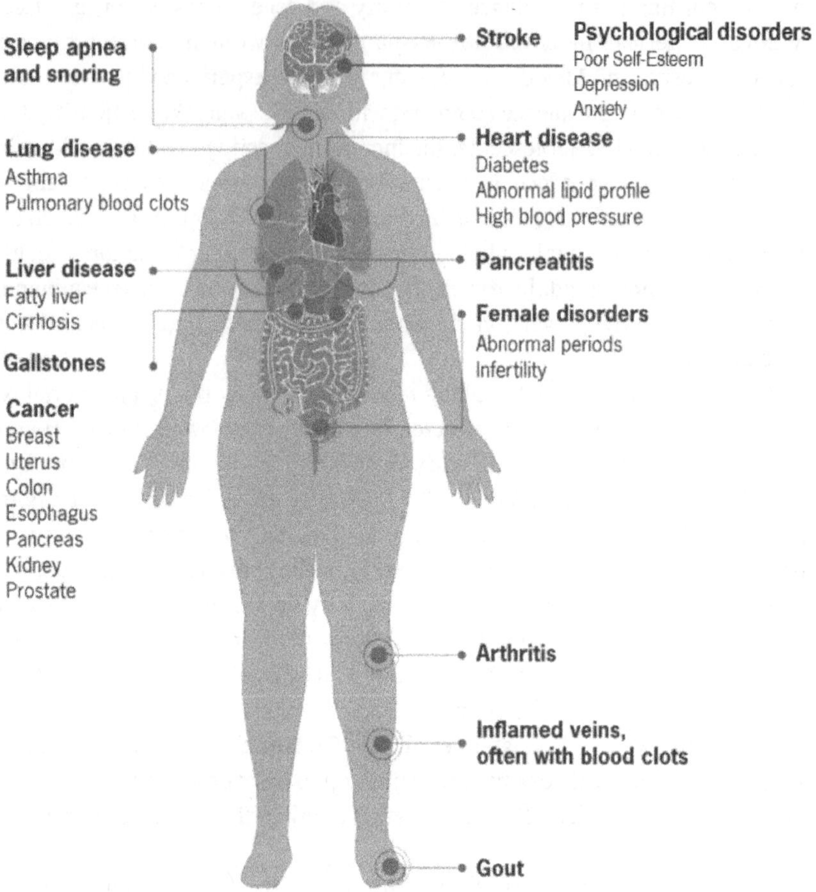

Sleep apnea and snoring

Lung disease
Asthma
Pulmonary blood clots

Liver disease
Fatty liver
Cirrhosis

Gallstones

Cancer
Breast
Uterus
Colon
Esophagus
Pancreas
Kidney
Prostate

Stroke

Psychological disorders
Poor Self-Esteem
Depression
Anxiety

Heart disease
Diabetes
Abnormal lipid profile
High blood pressure

Pancreatitis

Female disorders
Abnormal periods
Infertility

Arthritis

Inflamed veins, often with blood clots

Gout

Note. Adapted from the U.S. Centers for Disease Control and Prevention (2012).

continue to increase in the coming decades. In fact, estimates predict that by 2030 more than half of the adult population in the United States will have obesity and the prevalence of obesity in youth will have doubled (Y. Wang et al., 2008). Thus, it is likely psychologists and other mental health providers working in various settings will be tasked with providing prevention and treatment strategies and addressing psychological factors that influence the development and maintenance of obesity in youth.

PSYCHOLOGISTS' ROLE IN PREVENTION AND TREATMENT OF PEDIATRIC OBESITY

In 2007, the American Academy of Pediatrics published expert treatment recommendations, as well as staged treatment, for the prevention and assessment of pediatric obesity (Barlow & The Expert Committee, 2007). Staged treatment begins with Stage 1 (Prevention Plus), which focuses on promoting healthy eating and physical activity in youth diagnosed with overweight and related health risks or youth diagnosed with obesity. This treatment could occur in a primary care pediatric clinic. It continues through Stages 2 and 3 (Structured Weight Management and Comprehensive Multidisciplinary Intervention, respectively) to Stage 4 (Tertiary Care Intervention), which consists of youth diagnosed with severe obesity receiving care in a pediatric weight management center in which an interdisciplinary team provides comprehensive treatment ranging from very-low-calorie diets, to medications, to weight loss surgery. These recommendations were then updated in 2023 as clinical practice guidelines specific to evaluating and treating youth with obesity (Hampl et al., 2023a). Given the medical complexity related to the development and maintenance of excess weight in youth and its affect on major organ systems, the initial expert panel recommended comprehensive medical assessments and evaluation of weight-related medical issues in pediatric primary care settings when children have a BMI percentile in the overweight range (≥ the 85th percentile; Barlow & The Expert Committee, 2007). The medically recommended assessment and screening includes weight status assessment (e.g., BMI calculation); parental and family history of obesity and type 2 diabetes; and medical assessments specific to sleep problems, breathing problems, gastrointestinal issues, endocrine disorders, cardiovascular disorders, nervous system disorders, orthopedic issues, skin conditions, and genetic syndromes (Barlow & The Expert Committee, 2007). Vitals (heart rate, blood pressure) and other laboratory blood tests to assess for obesity-related comorbidities should also be implemented (Hampl et al., 2023a).

Social determinants of health are also critical components to include in assessment and screenings conducted for pediatric obesity and related comorbidities (Hampl et al., 2023a). Examples of social determinants of health that behavioral health providers should consider include "policies and systems, institutions and organizations (e.g., schools), neighborhoods and communities, and family, socioeconomic, environmental, ecological, genetic, and biological factors" (Hampl et al., 2023b, p. 2). Screening for psychiatric issues, such as depression, anxiety, eating disorders, and trauma, are also recommended in the pediatric primary care setting (Barlow & The Expert Committee, 2007). Pediatricians, other health care providers, and psychologists in a primary care setting would be appropriate providers to screen for these potential symptoms and social determinants of health. The most recent clinical practice guidelines also specifically state that motivational interviewing should be used by pediatricians and other health care providers to engage and treat youth with overweight and obesity and their families (Hampl et al., 2023a). As experts in understanding thoughts and behaviors, as well as trained informally and formally in motivational interviewing, psychologists and other mental health professionals are often involved in assisting with weight management efforts (American Psychological Association [APA], 2013). Psychologists are involved clinically in pediatric obesity prevention and treatment in various settings, such as specialty medical clinics, integrated primary care settings, and private practice. As experts in behavior change strategies, psychologists play an important role in the context of interdisciplinary care (APA, 2013). In interdisciplinary specialty care settings, such as pediatric weight management programs comprising clinicians from multiple disciplines (e.g., consistent with Stage 3 and Stage 4 treatment described by Barlow & The Expert Committee, 2007), mental health providers assess the child's and family's psychosocial environment and psychological concerns (APA, 2013). Specific constructs that psychologists should assess and consider in these settings are listed in Table 1.1. Assessments of these various constructs can range from unstructured to semistructured interviews to domain-specific questionnaires. Table 1.1 also provides examples of questionnaires or assessments that can assess specific constructs in pediatric obesity prevention and treatment settings. The use of specific standardized questionnaires should be determined on the basis of the setting and specific time- and funding-related limitations given that copyrighted questionnaires often have costs associated with both purchasing the questionnaire and scoring them. Other psychosocial factors that should be included in assessments include school functioning, social functioning, peer relationships (e.g., bullying, peer victimization), family relationships,

TABLE 1.1. Areas Psychologists Should Assess in Prevention and Treatment Settings for Pediatric Obesity

Construct	Example questionnaires/assessments	Reporter
Eating behaviors	Questionnaire of Eating and Weight Patterns-5 (Yanovski et al., 2015)	Self
Feeding behaviors	Parent Feeding Questionnaire (Kaur et al., 2006)	Caregiver
	Children's Eating Behaviour Questionnaire (Wardle et al., 2001)	Caregiver
Food selectivity and availability	Children's Eating Behaviour Questionnaire (Wardle et al., 2001)	Caregiver
	U.S. Household Food Security Survey Module (Tanaka et al., 2020)	Caregiver
Maladaptive/ disordered eating	Children's Eating Attitude Test (Maloney et al., 1988)	Self
Physical activity	Physical Activity Questionnaire for Older Children (Crocker et al., 1997)	Self
Sedentary behavior	Adolescent Sedentary Activity Questionnaire (Hardy et al., 2007)	Self
Sleep	Epworth Sleepiness Scale for Children and Adolescents (Johns, 2015)	Self
Psychological concerns		
Internalizing symptoms	Child Behavior Checklist (Achenbach & Rescorla, 2001)	• Self • Caregiver • Teacher
	Behavior Assessment Scale for Children (Reynolds & Kamphaus, 2015)	• Self • Caregiver • Teacher
Depressive symptoms	Patient Health Questionnaire-9 (Kroenke et al., 2001)	Self
Anxiety symptoms	General Anxiety Disorder-7 (Spitzer et al., 2006)	Self
Externalizing symptoms	Child Behavior Checklist (Achenbach & Rescorla, 2001)	• Self • Caregiver • Teacher
	Behavior Assessment Scale for Children (Reynolds & Kamphaus, 2015)	• Self • Caregiver • Teacher
ADHD or ODD symptoms	Vanderbilt ADHD Diagnostic Rating Scale (Wolraich et al., 2003)	Caregiver

Note. This table was created on the basis of information from the American Psychological Association (2013) and Cadieux et al. (2016). ADHD = attention-deficit/hyperactivity disorder; ODD = oppositional defiant disorder.

self-esteem, body image, motivation or readiness to change, and family support for changes (APA, 2013; Cadieux et al., 2016).

In addition to assessment, psychologists' role in interdisciplinary specialty care settings involves implementing behavioral components of weight management treatments that focus on dietary intake, physical activity, sleep, and other health behaviors associated with weight gain or lack of weight loss. These components may include monitoring lifestyle behaviors (e.g., eating and drinking, physical activity), increasing awareness regarding thoughts, feelings, and behaviors that are specifically related to food and eating or physical activity, and developing new skills to help modify lifestyle behaviors (APA, 2013). Specific psychological techniques and strategies related to behavioral components of pediatric weight management treatments are discussed in more detail in Part II of this book.

Psychologists provide treatment for specific psychological disorders in various settings treating patients with pediatric obesity. In primary care and interdisciplinary care settings, the treating psychologist should have knowledge, experience, and skills related to evidence-based treatments for psychological disorders with which children and adolescents with obesity may present. The application of specific evidence-based treatments in pediatric obesity are described in Part III of this book. Psychologists should also ensure that their treatment approaches and those of other health care providers are tailored to meet the specific needs of the child and family. In fact, the APA clinical practice panel for the treatment of overweight and obesity in children and adolescents "strongly recommends that providers be educated about the genetic, biological, psychological, social, and environmental complexities associated with obesity" (APA, 2018, p. 36). Bronfenbrenner's (1979) ecological model and bioecological theory (Bronfenbrenner, 1995) may be helpful frameworks. The ecological model purports that an individual's environment is divided into nested and interrelated systems (Ashiabi & O'Neal, 2015): the microsystem, mesosystem, exosystem, and macrosystem. The *microsystem* is the child's immediate environment and includes family, peers, and the school setting. The *mesosystem* involves interrelationships between different microsystems, and the *exosystem* is the setting in which the individual does not actively participate but has indirect effects on an individual's functioning. The *macrosystem* involves society and includes cultural values and economic conditions. Interrelations among the nested environments lead to patterns of interactions within these systems, which influence each other and affect individual outcomes (Bronfenbrenner, 1979). The bioecological model posits that reciprocal interactions occur between the person and the external environment for extended periods of time during development (Bronfenbrenner, 1995; see Figure 1.3).

Pediatric psychologists have applied both the bioecological and biopsychosocial models to health behaviors in youth; specifically, Wilson and Lawman (2009) reviewed research examining health promotion strategies implemented in microsystems (families, peers), mesosystems (schools), exosystems (communities, mass media), and macrosystems (public policies). Other models have been developed to incorporate cultural and diversity-related factors, such as the African American Collaborative Obesity Research Network model (Kumanyika et al., 2007), which has broader implications for the prevention and treatment of obesity and obesity-related health disparities and can apply to other racial/ethnic and marginalized groups.

In 2015, The Obesity Society developed an infographic to represent contributors to obesity identified by previous research (The Obesity Society, 2015). In the figure, which visually represents the complexity of obesity, the potential causes of obesity are divided as occurring inside and outside the person (see Figure 4.1 for an adapted version of the figure).

FIGURE 1.3. The Bioecological Model

Social and health systems, policies, laws, cultural values and beliefs

Neighborhood safety and resources, school district, mass media

Parent workplace and policies, skilled educators and providers

Home environment, parent mental health, parenting, family relationships

Social, economic and cultural contexts and policies

Neighborhoods and communities

Supportive school, work, and religious settings

Parent & family well-being

Child & youth well-being and resilience

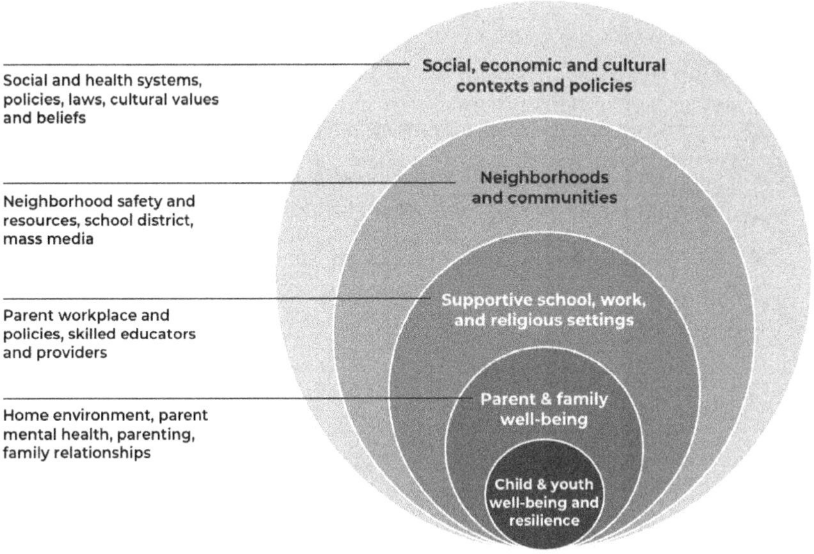

Note. From *The Bioecological Model*, by the Center for Child & Family Well-Being, University of Washington, 2021 (https://ccfwb.uw.edu/about-us/the-bioecological-model/). Copyright 2021 by the Center for Child & Family Well-Being. Reprinted with permission.

Given the complexities regarding the development, treatment, and intractability of pediatric obesity, we hope this book will be a helpful resource for current and future psychologists, trainees, and other mental health care providers working in various settings to prevent and treat obesity in youth and families while addressing psychological factors from a multicultural and diversity, equity, and inclusion lens.

CONCLUSION

Pediatric obesity is both a significant public health concern and a serious chronic health condition. The prevention and treatment of pediatric obesity require knowledge regarding psychological factors; social determinants of health, and diversity, equity, and inclusion issues that are associated with the development of obesity and may affect treatment strategies. This book is intended to be an evidence-based resource regarding these topics, one that is based on available research and clinical experience, for psychologists and other mental health providers working in settings focused on the prevention and treatment of pediatric obesity.

KEY POINTS

- Pediatric obesity is a complex chronic medical condition.
- Psychological factors, social determinants of health, and health disparity and health equity issues are important factors that must be considered.
- Psychologists and other behavioral health specialists play an important role in the prevention and treatment of this condition.

THINKING OUTSIDE THE BOX

What are arguments for and against diagnosing obesity on the basis of BMI?

2 HEALTH EQUITY, HEALTH DISPARITIES, AND DIVERSITY

Despite a trend of stabilizing obesity rates over the past decade (Hales et al., 2017), children and adolescents from certain backgrounds continue to experience disproportionate rates of obesity (Ogden et al., 2020). Contributing to this disproportionality are a number of complex social and environmental factors that interact with genetic and biological mechanisms (Browne et al., 2022). It is critical that clinicians, researchers, and policymakers acknowledge systemic racism, economic disparities, cultural differences, and social determinants of health in their efforts to address pediatric obesity (Kumanyika, 2019; Mackey et al., 2022). For example, traditional measures of obesity (i.e., body mass index [BMI]) may not be applicable across racial/ethnic groups, and typical nutrition recommendations may not be attainable for families experiencing food insecurity.

The purpose of this chapter is to highlight issues of health equity, health disparities, and cultural diversity as they relate to the psychological treatment of pediatric obesity (see Table 2.1). According to the U. S. Centers for

https://doi.org/10.1037/0000401-002
Psychological Approaches to the Treatment of Pediatric Obesity, by C. S. Lim and E. T. Burton

TABLE 2.1. Diversity Terms and Pediatric Obesity Examples

Term	Definition	Example
Health equity	The fair and just attainment of full health potential for all individuals. Attaining health equity requires systems-level change to acknowledge current and past injustices, address social and economic barriers to health and health care, and eliminate health disparities.	The mayor of a city allocates funding to the department of parks and recreation to update facilities at each playground in the city. When the updates are completed, each household in the city has access to a safe and functional playground within a 1 mile (1.6 km) vicinity.
Health disparities	Preventable and unjust inequities in the quality of health, access to health care, and health outcomes that are linked to social, economic, and/or environmental disadvantage.	Taylor lives in a state whose Medicaid program does not cover Wegovy, an effective weight loss medication. Taylor's family cannot afford the out-of-pocket cost of more than $1,000/month for the medication, so Taylor is prescribed a less effective medication.
Cultural diversity	Differences in beliefs, values, behaviors, and response patterns influenced by an individual and group identity and characteristics (e.g., language, race/ethnicity, religious beliefs, sexual orientation, nationality, social background).	Kai is a transgender young woman who wants to play basketball for her high school. Because of school policy, she is not allowed to use the girl's locker room and is banned from joining the girls' basketball team. Joining the boys' team is not consistent with her gender identity, which leaves Kai with no opportunity to engage in the exercise she enjoys.
Cultural humility	Awareness, acknowledgment, and appreciation that one will never be fully competent in the understanding of how cultural differences influence others' experiences; a lifelong commitment to self-critique, self-evaluation, and openness to learning from others.	Staff at a pediatric weight management clinic attend an annual retreat where they examine their own biases and hear from speakers who share their lived experiences with obesity.

TABLE 2.1. Diversity Terms and Pediatric Obesity Examples (*Continued*)

Term	Definition	Example
Systemic racism	Systems-level (e.g., legal, political, educational, health care) practices, policies, norms, rules, and laws that uphold, maintain, and reinforce race-based inequities, oppression, and unjust treatment. Racism can be conscious or unconscious, intentional, or unintentional, explicit or implicit. In a health context, these systems and structures impede the pursuit of good health and well-being by people of color. *Systemic racism* is often used synonymously with *structural* and *institutional racism*.	Quentin, a Black father of two children, was sentenced to 10 years in prison for a minor drug crime. Although his lawyer argued that this sentence was excessive, the judge was not swayed. While Quentin is incarcerated, his family faces financial struggles and food insecurity. Limited access to healthy foods contributes to his children's weight gain and insulin resistance.
Social determinants of health	Environmental factors that contribute to health disparities, health functioning, and quality of life. These determinants are grouped into five domains: 1. Economic stability 2. Education access and quality 3. Health care access and quality 4. Neighborhood and built environment 5. Social and community context	Paloma is a 17-year-old who lives in a rural community that is 3 hours away from the nearest academic medical center. Although she is referred for bariatric surgery to treat her severe obesity and hypertension, her mother is unable to take the time off work to transport Paloma to monthly appointments with the bariatric clinic.

Note. This table was created on the basis of information from Braveman et al. (2022), Egede et al. (2023), Gómez et al. (2021), and Mackey et al. (2022).

Disease Control and Prevention (CDC; 2022b), health equity is achieved when everyone has a fair and just opportunity to be as healthy as possible. This entails addressing barriers that prevent individuals and communities from reaching their highest level of health. It is important to note that equity is not the same as equality. A useful example to discern the concepts is to consider a group of high school students being provided uniforms for their school's sports teams. *Equality* would be providing each young person exactly the same type and size uniform—a size medium t-shirt and shorts. In line with the theme of this chapter, however, we know that there is tremendous diversity in terms of adolescents' body shapes and sizes, and they have different needs depending on unique circumstances. Therefore, *equity* would be checking in with each adolescent to see what they need to be successful. A soccer player of medium build may thrive in the t-shirt and shorts. However, an ice hockey player living in a larger body will have more difficulty excelling at their sport without considering their specific need for helmet, gloves, pads, and skates.

The pursuit of health equity requires elimination of preventable *health disparities*, which are differences in individuals' health status related to sociodemographic factors such as race/ethnicity, socioeconomic status (SES), and geographic region. Furthermore, the pursuit of health equity requires a culturally humble approach that acknowledges the diverse identities of children, adolescents, and families with obesity (Kibakaya & Oyeku, 2022; Tervalon & Murray-García, 1998).

RACE/ETHNICITY

Although the prevalence of obesity among U.S. children and adolescents is 19.3%, rates are disproportionately higher among youth identifying as American Indian/Alaska Native (29.7%), Hispanic (25.6%), and non-Hispanic Black (24.2%; Bullock et al., 2017; Fryar et al., 2020). These disparities in pediatric obesity are attributable, in part, to a long and ingrained history of racism and discrimination in the United States. Systemic discrimination and racism contribute to limited educational opportunities, economic disadvantage, and inequitable access to health care, all of which exacerbate disparate health outcomes (Mackey et al., 2022; Neblett, 2019). Of recent note, the disproportionate toll the COVID-19 pandemic has taken on communities of color highlights the myriad health disparities affecting youth from historically marginalized backgrounds (Hooper et al., 2020).

In addition to disproportionate obesity prevalence, youth of color also experience disparities in terms of assessment and access to evidence-based obesity treatment. Current CDC growth curves, which define body mass index percentiles, were developed using data from mostly White children and do not account for racial/ethnic differences in body composition and fat distribution (Freedman et al., 2008). Failure to acknowledge such differences can lead to inaccurate obesity classifications, inappropriate screening for comorbidities, and misguided treatment recommendations. Relatedly, *implicit bias*—unconscious negative stereotypes, attitudes, and perceptions toward a specific social group—can play a role in treatment planning and referral patterns for youth of color.

Several studies have revealed the presence of implicit bias among health care workers, including physicians, nurses, and psychologists (FitzGerald & Hurst, 2017; T. J. Johnson et al., 2017; Ricks et al., 2022). Guedj and colleagues (2021) found, in a sample of pediatric emergency physicians, that participants displayed implicit bias against Hispanic and non-Hispanic Black individuals as well as individuals with obesity. These biases were correlated, suggesting that some physicians may have multiple and overlapping biases. Such biases may be related to the underutilization of evidence-based obesity treatment options by youth of color, including metabolic and bariatric surgery (Perez et al., 2020). Recent findings suggest that explicitly targeting pediatric obesity-related biases through educational interventions is effective and worthwhile (Rincon-Subtirelu, 2017).

A final consideration for the role of race/ethnicity in pediatric obesity are cultural beliefs and practices. Factors such as parental feeding style, food and beverage preferences, and body image all have strong linkages to culture and weight outcomes (Kumanyika, 2008). For example, forcing children to continue eating when they are no longer hungry may have roots in tradition, an authoritarian parenting style, past or recurring economic hardship, or misperception of a child's weight. Such behaviors can eventually override innate appetite regulation mechanisms (J. O. Fisher & Kral, 2008). Likewise, cultural perceptions of health relative to body size can contribute to pediatric obesity. Research on weight perception and body satisfaction reveals that Hispanic and non-Hispanic Black individuals tend to report larger ideal body sizes (Killion et al., 2006; S. H. Thompson et al., 1997). Similarly, youth of color with obesity and their caregivers have been shown to underestimate their weight, making them less amenable to weight management guidance (Blanchet et al., 2019; Ling & Stommel, 2019). It is important to note, however, that weight misperception has been found to be protective in terms of depression, disordered eating, and future weight gain (Sonneville et al., 2016; Thurston et al., 2017). Recent literature suggests that the potential protection of weight misperception may be driven by strong racial identity and racial socialization (Lisse et al., 2022).

SOCIOECONOMIC STATUS

The current literature suggests that racial/ethnic disparities in pediatric obesity are driven largely by disparities in socioeconomic status (SES; Fradkin et al., 2015; Vazquez & Cubbin, 2020). Youth from lower SES backgrounds are more likely to have obesity than their more affluent counterparts. However, higher income is less protective for Hispanic and non-Hispanic Black children compared with non-Hispanic White children (Assari, 2018).

Examinations of environmental factors have revealed that communities with limited access to grocery stores offering healthy foods and safe spaces for physical activity have higher rates of pediatric obesity (Cobb et al., 2015; Malacarne et al., 2022). Put more specifically, youth living in neighborhoods with greater access to convenience stores are more likely to develop obesity (Ohri-Vachaspati et al., 2021), and youth living in closer proximity to recreational resources are less likely to gain excess weight (Wolch et al., 2011). Again, from a systemic perspective, children and families from racially/ethnically minoritized backgrounds are more likely to live in lower income neighborhoods and in turn are more likely to have limited options for healthy food and physical activity. Oftentimes, the educational, occupational, and economic disadvantage that is common in lower SES environments is generational and determined by years of systemic racism and discrimination (Bailey et al., 2017; Mackey et al., 2022).

The above-mentioned findings underscore the importance of taking a more nuanced view of systemic inequities that make certain youth more vulnerable to obesity and its comorbidities. For example, L. Brown and colleagues (2015) conducted qualitative interviews with caregivers of children with overweight and obesity and reported a number of perceived barriers to weight management, including inadequate financial resources for physical activities, limited access to exercise programming, limited time to prepare healthy meals and exercise with their children, and lack of knowledge regarding healthy behaviors for their children. Conversely, a higher education level of the head of the household is associated with more robust protection against pediatric obesity for youth from a variety of racial/ethnic backgrounds (Ogden et al., 2018).

GEOGRAPHIC REGION

Children and families living in rural communities are at greater risk of over-weight and obesity than those living in more urban environments (J. A. Johnson & Johnson, 2015). Not only do these medically underresourced areas have a lower patient-to-primary care physician ratio, but also rural residents may experience greater transportation difficulties because they may need to travel long distances to reach health care facilities (Hing & Hsiao, 2014). Additional barriers include limited economic resources, limited access to healthy food options, a lack of safe spaces devoted to physical activity, and cultural beliefs and practices (Janicke et al., 2019; C. S. Lim & Janicke, 2013). In terms of pediatric weight management, comprehensive interdisciplinary treatment programs tend to be affiliated with academic medical centers, which are less prevalent in rural communities (Findholt et al., 2013).

INTERSECTIONALITY

As discussed, individuals possess multiple identities that influence their health status and access to health resources. Unfortunately, research and clinical practice have tended to isolate identities, neglecting the inherent nuance of lived experiences as affected by multiple and complex inter-secting identities. The intersectionality framework highlights how societal structures of oppression, marginalization, and exclusion work together to maintain health disparities (Bowleg, 2012). The interaction of socio-demographic factors (e.g., race/ethnicity, SES, geographic region) with obesity cannot be unraveled and should not be considered separately. Behavioral health specialists are especially well positioned to take a more holistic view of how the intersection of systemic factors and lived experience contribute to obesity-related health outcomes in children, adolescents, and families.

CONCLUSION

Pediatric obesity is a complex condition that is influenced by many factors besides biology, genetics, and conscious behavior. The sociodemographic factors reviewed in this chapter represent only a sampling of the unique experiences children and families face that place them at greater risk for obesity and its comorbidities. The treatment approaches discussed in this book require a lens through which to view disparities and inequities as well as the intersectionality of pediatric obesity and diverse identities.

KEY POINTS

- Achieving equity in terms of pediatric obesity-related health outcomes requires multiple levels of action.

- Psychologists and behavioral health specialists can serve as drivers of taking an intersectional approach to the treatment of pediatric obesity.

THINKING OUTSIDE THE BOX

What are some actionable strategies that can be implemented to improve equitable access to healthy resources?

3 WEIGHT-RELATED STIGMA AND DISCRIMINATION

In addition to the physiological consequences associated with pediatric obesity, children and adolescents with excess weight are more likely than their normal-weight peers to experience psychosocial distress (Burton, Jones, et al., 2020; Pulgarón, 2013). In particular, these youth are more susceptible to weight-based victimization, including teasing, bullying, discrimination, and stigma (Puhl & Latner, 2007). Perceived or experienced weight stigma is a chronic stressor for many youth and is associated with adverse mental health outcomes (Emmer et al., 2020). Unfortunately, pediatric weight management prevention and intervention efforts often fail to acknowledge or address this serious issue. Considering the strong evidence linking weight stigma to increased vulnerability for depression, anxiety, low self-esteem, poor body image, substance use, and suicidality among youth, more attention by clinicians, researchers, and policymakers is critical (Pont et al., 2017; Puhl & Lessard, 2020).

https://doi.org/10.1037/0000401-003
Psychological Approaches to the Treatment of Pediatric Obesity, by C. S. Lim and E. T. Burton

WHAT IS WEIGHT STIGMA?

Stigma generally refers to negative beliefs and attitudes, disapproval of, or discrimination against an individual or group that influence interactions in a detrimental way. *Weight stigma*, therefore, is devaluation of an individual with overweight or obesity (Pont et al., 2017). Stigma manifests in many forms, including verbal (e.g., insults, derogatory names, pejorative language), physical (e.g., touching, grabbing), and relational (e.g., ostracization, rejection, being the subject of rumors). Moreover, weight stigma influences stereotypes that individuals with obesity are lazy, unmotivated, or undisciplined (Puhl & Lessard, 2020). Such stereotypes are dangerous in that they can lead to unjust treatment, prejudice, and discrimination. Although stigma and discrimination are generally considered to be counter to the ideals of diversity, equity, and inclusion, weight stigma tends to be more tolerated than stigma that is based on gender, race/ethnicity, or age (Puhl, Andreyeva, & Brownell, 2008). Put more specifically, weight stigma has been identified as "the last socially acceptable form of prejudice" (Budd et al., 2011, p. 136).

Weight stigma often stems from beliefs that shame will motivate individuals to lose weight (Palad et al., 2019). In fact, stigmatizing words and actions may be intended as encouragement to lead to engagement in healthier behaviors. However, research reveals that weight stigma can actually lead to behaviors such as binge eating, decreased physical activity, and social isolation, thereby worsening obesity and creating additional barriers to healthy behavior change (Pont et al., 2017). A prospective study of middle and high school students found that weight-based teasing was a significant predictor of disordered eating behaviors (Haines et al., 2006), and many researchers have found that weight stigma impairs overall quality of life (Puhl & Lessard, 2020). Of significant concern is that weight stigma may cause individuals to internalize their negative experiences, a phenomenon termed *weight bias internalization* (Puhl et al., 2018). Although internalized weight bias is not well studied in children and adolescents, youth who report experiencing higher rates of teasing and lower self-esteem seem to be more likely to accept and agree to negative descriptors of themselves—and apply these negative inferences to themselves (Fields et al., 2021; Tanas et al., 2022). Overall, weight stigma impedes progress in effectively addressing obesity prevention and intervention, in particular among youth (Kyle et al., 2018).

For youth with obesity, weight stigma most often tends to take the forms of teasing and bullying. Early research on the topic found that 63% of girls and 58% of boys with obesity reported being teased about their weight (Neumark-Sztainer et al., 2002). More contemporary findings suggest that weight-based teasing is becoming even more common, with up to 71% of youth reporting weight-based teasing and bullying (Puhl et al., 2013). Although weight-based stigma seems to occur most often in the school environment, youth are victimized across multiple settings. Peers, educators, family members, health care professionals, and society at large have all been reported to engage in weight stigma (Puhl & Heuer, 2010).

Weight Stigma in the Educational Setting

Children and adolescents spend a considerable amount of their time in school environments, and previous studies have shown that youth report experiencing weight-based teasing most often in the school setting (I. Thompson et al., 2020). In fact, youth with obesity experience significantly more teasing and bullying overall, whether or not related to weight and regardless of race/ethnicity, family income, and academic achievement (Krukowski et al., 2008; Lumeng et al., 2010).

There is evidence that children experience weight-based teasing early on, even as young as age 3 to 4 years, highlighting a need for early anti-bias intervention (Cramer & Steinwert, 1998; Ruffman et al., 2016). Palad and colleagues (2019) pointed out that in addition to the acute embarrassment and sadness that children and adolescents experience in relation to teasing and bullying, the chronic accumulation of these negative experiences in their daily life affects their overall quality of life.

In addition to weight-based teasing within peer relationships, weight stigma can present in many other ways in the school environment. Data reveal that in terms of social, physical, and academic skills, educators have lower expectations for their students with obesity compared with students without obesity (Greenleaf et al., 2008; Nutter et al., 2019; Zavodny, 2013). Furthermore, teachers have been shown to endorse stereotypical assumptions that students with excess weight are not as intelligent, competent, successful, or hard working as their peers with normal weight (Puhl & Heuer, 2009). Unfortunately, such biases may lead to weight-related gaps in educational attainment and achievement (Lessard & Puhl, 2021).

A less researched aspect of weight stigma in the school setting is appropriate and comfortable physical accommodations. For example, standard-sized desks, playground equipment, and bathroom stalls can present a painful and humiliating experience for some youth with obesity (Beck, 2016). Solutions such as having a child sit at a table while other students sit in desks, or wear different clothing when school uniforms are not available in larger sizes, can be embarrassing and provide another target for teasing and bullying.

Advocating for a more inclusive physical environment can reduce weight stigma and discrimination in the school setting.

Weight Stigma in the Familial Environment

Like the educational setting, the familial environment plays a significant role in child development. Family-based weight stigma can manifest as teasing, name-calling, exclusion, or hostility, and researchers suggest that the consequences may be more negative and enduring for youth than weight stigma by nonfamilial sources (Hunger & Tomiyama, 2018; Lawrence et al., 2022). Weight stigma expressed by caregivers has been shown to influence emotional well-being through adulthood (Puhl, Moss-Racusin, et al., 2008). In fact, participants in a qualitative study of adults with obesity attributed their most "significant stigmatizing event" to weight-related comments from their parents (Vartanian et al., 2014). It is important to note that family-based weight stigma is promulgated by other family members as well, most notably siblings (Berge et al., 2016).

In line with the assertion that stigmatizing comments regarding weight are intended to be motivating, qualitative accounts from family members revealed that weight-oriented talk often is rooted in concerns about health and well-being (Berge, Trofholz, et al., 2015). This same study also reported that family members teased their children about weight to protect them from hurtful comments from others outside the family. This does not negate the deleterious effects of weight stigma (Lessard et al., 2021).

Another important aspect of weight stigma in the family environment is the experience of *stigma by association* (Gorlick et al., 2021), which is a phenomenon in which an individual is stigmatized because of someone else's stigmatized condition. In the case of pediatric obesity, studies have found that caregivers may feel shamed and guilted by criticisms of their parenting behaviors that may contribute to excess weight (K. M. Lee et al., 2022). This is particularly prominent among caregivers who report being questioned about their feeding practices by health care professionals (Gorlick et al., 2021).

Weight Stigma in Health Care Settings

One of the most troubling consequences of weight stigma in youth with obesity is avoidance of the health care system (Mensinger et al., 2018). At baseline, patients with obesity are less likely to obtain preventative health services such as annual physical exams and cancer screenings (Alberga et al., 2019). In addition, research shows that when patients encounter stigmatizing interactions with health care professionals (including physicians, nurses, psychologists, and dietitians), they are even more likely to delay or cancel appointments (Tomiyama et al., 2018).

Evaluations of health care professionals' weight biases have revealed implicit associations of obesity with poor adherence, dishonesty, laziness, lower intelligence, and lack of self-control (Puhl & Heuer, 2009; Sabin et al., 2012). Perhaps because of these assumptions, health care professionals have been found to spend less time with patients with obesity; be less willing to treat patients who are obese; and attribute health concerns to patients' weight, despite viable alternate explanations (Tomiyama et al., 2018). As a result, patients report feeling ignored, undervalued, and mistreated by their clinicians (Rathbone et al., 2023). Figure 3.1 illustrates how negative

FIGURE 3.1. The Cycle of Weight Stigma and Obesity

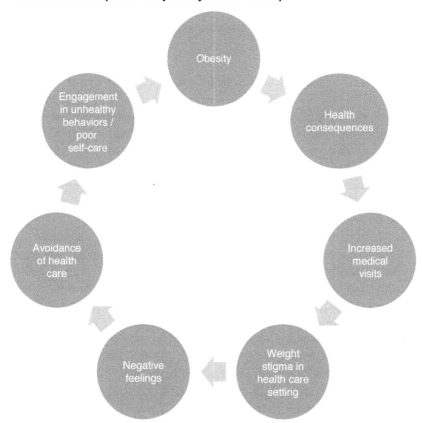

Note. This figure created on the basis of information presented in Puhl & Heuer (2009).

interactions with the health care system can lead to worse obesity-related health outcomes. Children experiencing weight-related bias and stigma tend to report poorer mental health outcomes (Warnick et al., 2022), which underscores the crucial role of behavioral health specialists in addressing pediatric obesity. Clinicians are encouraged to be thoughtful of how they discuss weight with youth, bearing in mind the risk of disengagement with treatment and exacerbation of physiological and mental health outcomes.

In addition to interpersonal concerns in the health care setting, patients also report weight stigma and discrimination in terms of barriers, obstacles, and physical accommodations. For example, waiting room chairs, exam tables, patient gowns, and medical equipment (e.g., blood pressure cuffs and scales that do not accommodate bodies of larger size) contribute to a less welcoming clinical environment and diminishes the quality of health care that is provided (Palad et al., 2019; Pont et al., 2017).

WHAT CAN HEALTH CARE PROVIDERS DO TO COMBAT WEIGHT STIGMA?

The origins of weight stigma likely lie in oversimplified attributions about the causes of obesity. For example, the Energy Balance Model (see Figure 3.2) suggests that weight control is as straightforward as "calories in, calories out." As researchers have developed a more complex understanding of obesity, the Energy Balance Model now reflects endocrine, metabolic, and nervous system signals that interact with environmental influences (see Hall et al., 2022). Nevertheless, the more simplified model continues to perpetuate the idea that obesity is a personal failing that is easily reversible if one tries hard enough.

Weight stigma is also perpetuated in popular media. Multiple studies have shown that television programs and movies targeting younger audiences often negatively portray characters with obesity in stereotypical roles (i.e., unattractive, unappealing, shown eating or overeating, as the target of jokes or cruelty; Palad et al., 2019; Pont et al., 2017). Furthermore, media targeting children rarely acknowledge the harmful outcomes of unhealthy eating and sedentary behaviors, which may lead viewers to engage in similar behaviors with no expectation of negative consequences (Eisenberg et al., 2015; Howard et al., 2017). Even health education campaigns to address pediatric obesity have been shown to incorporate weight-stigmatizing imagery (Pearl et al., 2015). Using an experimental design, Pearl and colleagues (2012) found that positive portrayals of individuals with obesity in the media can actually help reduce weight stigma.

FIGURE 3.2. The Energy Balance Model of Obesity: Oversimplification of a Complex Condition

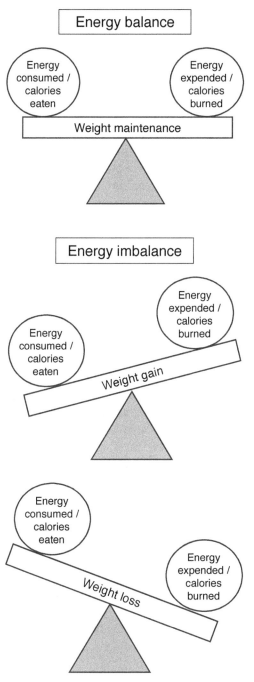

In recent years, several prominent health care organizations and associations have made similar calls to reduce and ultimately eliminate weight stigma. The World Health Organization Regional Office for Europe (2017) and American Academy of Pediatrics (Pont et al., 2017) have issued policy statements, and the following organizations partnered to develop a joint international consensus statement for ending obesity-related stigma (Rubino et al., 2020): American Association of Clinical Endocrinologists, American Society for Metabolic and Bariatric Surgery, American Diabetes Association, Diabetes UK, European Association for the Study of Obesity, International Federation for the Surgery of Obesity and Metabolic Disorders, Obesity Action Coalition, Obesity Canada, The Obesity Society, and World Obesity Federation. Each of these statements acknowledges that weight stigma contributes to poor health and impairs appropriate treatment. However, in order to see reduction and elimination of weight stigma, these statements must be implemented and executed in a meaningful way. There is still much work to be done.

CONCLUSION

Unlike other forms of discrimination, such as gender, race/ethnicity, and age, there are few legal protections for weight-based stigma and discrimination. In fact, negative comments about weight are often presented as motivation and encouragement. At the time of this writing, Michigan is the only state with laws banning discrimination on the basis of body size, and New York City recently enacted legislation prohibiting height or weight discrimination in employment, housing, and public accommodations.

Considering the harms associated with weight bias, clinicians working with youth with obesity also have an important platform to model and advocate for unbiased and nondiscriminatory treatment. The following are some specific recommendations to help health care professionals, including psychologists and behavioral health specialists, combat weight stigma (Puhl, 2013):

- Anticipate that you will see patients with obesity.
- Be mindful of patients' previous negative experiences.
- Recognize the multiple factors that contribute to overweight and obesity.
- Explore all causes of presentation, not just weight.
- Recognize that many patients have tried to lose weight.
- Emphasize the importance of behavior change.
- Acknowledge the difficulty of making lifestyle changes.
- Focus more on outcomes related to health and wellness and less on weight and shape.

KEY POINTS

- Weight bias and stigma occur in all environments and can be overt or covert.

- We encourage psychologists and behavioral health specialists to be mindful of how they discuss weight with youth, taking their lead in terms of terminology used.

THINKING OUTSIDE THE BOX

Is it possible to motivate youth with obesity to improve their health without engaging in bias or stigma?

4 ETIOLOGY OF PEDIATRIC OBESITY

Numerous factors influence the onset, maintenance, and intractability of obesity in youth. These range from genetic and biological causes to social and environmental factors. For children, the family environment also needs to be taken into account. Recognizing the intersectionality of these influences is also important to consider. In this chapter, we review research and clinical findings related to obesity-related causes and factors that psychologists and other medical and mental health providers should consider in the prevention and treatment of pediatric obesity.

Ecological and biopsychosocial models are helpful to conceptualize factors that may contribute to obesity development and maintenance. The Obesity Society (2015) developed an infographic on the basis of findings from a work group that reviewed research findings from various disciplines, which pictorially represents more than 100 potential factors associated with obesity and divides them into factors within the individual and those outside the individual (see Figure 4.1 for an adapted version).

https://doi.org/10.1037/0000401-004
Psychological Approaches to the Treatment of Pediatric Obesity, by C. S. Lim and E. T. Burton

FIGURE 4.1. Potential Contributors to Obesity

	Inside the Person	Outside the Person
Increased Intake	Biological/Medical[a] Psychological[b]	Biological/Medical[h] Food & beverage behavior/environment[i] Economic[j]
Intake & Expenditure	Maternal/Developmental[c] Biological/Medical[d] Psychological[e]	Maternal/Developmental[k] Biological/Medical[l] Psychological[m] Economic[n] Social[o] Environmental pressures on physical activity[p]
Decreased Expenditure	Biological/Medical[f] Psychological[g]	Maternal/Developmental[q] Environmental pressures on physical activity[r]

Contributors to Energy Storage

Note. Figure created on the basis of information presented by The Obesity Society (2015). Superscript letters denote specific examples of potential contributing factors. [a]Hyperreactivity to environmental food cues, heightened hunger response, delayed satiety; [b]Disordered eating, emotional coping; [c]Gestational diabetes; [d]Genetic and epigenetic factors, age-related changes, chronic inflammation, pathological sources of endocrine dysregulation, central and peripheral regulators of appetite and adipose tissue; [e]Self-regulatory and coping deficits, trauma history, mood disturbance, mental health concerns; [f]Thermogensis, gut microbiota, pain sensitivity, physical disabilities; [g]Social anxiety; [h]Environmental/chemical toxins; [i]Larger portion sizes, skipping meals, increased availability of high-calorie/high-sugar foods and drinks, food insecurity, eating away from home, lack of family meals, eating as recreation, snacking, and special occasions, lack of nutritional education; [j]Market economy, food surplus, pervasive food marketing; [k]Maternal employment, breastfeeding, maternal stress, maternal smoking, maternal obesity, delayed prenatal care, birth order, having children, nonparental child care, maternal over-nutrition during pregnancy, birth by c-section; [l]Infection, weight gain–inducing drugs, smoking cessation, sleep deficits; [m]Stress, child maltreatment, weight cycling; [n]Westernization and economic development, low socioeconomic status and nutrition support; [o]Family conflict, social networks, being in a romantic relationship, lack of employer ability to assist with obesity, weight bias and stigma, lack of health care provider support/knowledge and inadequate access to care; [p]Living in a crime-prone area; [q]Prenatal air pollution; [r]Temperature regulation, increased sedentary time, built environment, decreased opportunity for non-exercise–based physical activity, manual labor-saving devices.

GENETIC AND EPIGENETIC FACTORS

Previous research has estimated that adult body mass index (BMI) heritability is 73%, but estimates also vary widely, ranging from 31% to 90% (Min et al., 2013). More recent research with children has revealed that genetic factors accounted for 62% of the change in body mass index across a 4-year period (Schrempft et al., 2018). In general, genetic causes of obesity can be categorized into *monogenic causes*, or single gene mutations that disturb appetite; *syndromic causes*, characterized by severe obesity with other medical and developmental comorbidities; and *polygenic causes*, or the cumulative impact on a large number of genes (Thaker, 2017).

Leptin is the primary hormone involved in signaling a feeling of fullness. Most types of monogenic obesity are associated with mutations to the leptin gene or leptin receptor and are characterized by *hyperphagia*, or the lack of feeling full, that results in early-onset severe obesity (Thaker, 2017). Prevalence rates for leptin receptor mutations are estimated at 2% to 3% of the general population, and leptin gene mutations are considered even more rare (e.g., only a few dozen cases have been identified in the medical literature; Thaker, 2017).

There are numerous genetic syndromes associated with the development of obesity in youth. Prader–Willi, Bardet–Biedl, and Alström syndromes are examples of genetic conditions associated with obesity onset in early childhood. Prader–Willi syndrome has been linked to a specific genetic loci (e.g., 15q11–q13) and is perhaps most well known for hallmark symptoms of hyperphagia and insatiable appetite, as well as developmental delays and behavioral problems (Chung et al., 2020). It is estimated to occur in 1 in 15,000 to 25,000 births, and the life expectancy is about 30 years (Chung et al., 2020; J. L. Miller & Tan, 2020). Bardet–Biedl syndrome is an autosomal recessive disorder linked to multiple genetic loci and mutations (more than 16 disease-causing genes) and is estimated to affect 1 in 13,500 to 160,000 births (Forsythe & Beales, 2013). It is characterized by vision and kidney problems, as well as obesity and type 2 diabetes and developmental delays. Alström syndrome is also an autosomal recessive disorder and is caused by genetic mutations in ALMS1 (S. Kang, 2021). It is considered ultra rare, affecting 1 in 1,000,000 people (Dassie et al., 2021). Neurological, vision, kidney, and heart problems, as well as significant metabolic issues, characterize this syndrome. Research suggests that most individuals with Alström syndrome develop obesity by 5 years of age and eventually develop related medical comorbidities, such as insulin resistance and type 2 diabetes (S. Kang, 2021).

In order to diagnose these specific monogenic and syndromic conditions, genetic testing is necessary. In recent years, advances have been made that have increased access to and utilization of genetic testing to screen for potential genetic causes of obesity, and new genetic markers associated with obesity are rapidly being discovered (Rhythm Pharmaceuticals, 2021). The hope is that personalized medicine based on genetics will lead to targeted medical interventions. Until recently, no targeted pharmacological treatments were widely available for these genetic syndromes, but advances in genetic testing and increased knowledge regarding implicated genes have made possible the development of drug therapies that target genetic influences of obesity onset and maintenance. Lifestyle approaches targeting nutritional intake and physical activity remain the primary treatment for children with monogenic and syndromic forms of obesity.

Epigenetics has also been examined as a potential contributor to obesity development. Unlike the specific genetic syndromes just discussed, *epigenetics* refers to chemical modifications to DNA that are thought to be reversible and heritable (van Dijk et al., 2015). The most widely recognized impact is made by *methylation*, whereby methyl groups are added to DNA. There is evidence that exposure to various nutritional and environmental factors, such as under- or overexposure to nutrition prenatally and the resulting methylation, may lead to later development of obesity. In addition, in adults with obesity, interventions that focus on nutrition and physical activity, as well as weight loss surgery, influence methylation markers and result in profiles similar to those of adults without obesity. Research in this area with children and adolescents is limited; however, findings suggest that the interactions between genetics and the environment are important to consider and that pediatric obesity prevention efforts should target the prenatal environment. In addition, epigenetic factors should be examined during and after weight management treatment in adults and their future children.

Although genetics and epigenetics play a role in obesity etiology, these specifically identified causes of obesity are rare and together do not alone account for the sharp increase in obesity prevalence rates seen in recent decades.

OTHER BIOLOGICAL AND MEDICAL FACTORS

Numerous biological and medical factors have also been identified as related to causing initial weight gain, as well as to difficulties related to initiating and maintaining weight loss, which are important for pediatric psychologists and other medical providers to keep in mind when involved in pediatric obesity prevention and treatment efforts.

Inflammation in the body occurs in response to acute or chronic disruptions in cellular functioning and physiology, such as the presence of bacteria or specific environmental signals (Singer & Lumeng, 2017). Specific to obesity, inflammation can occur in response to overfeeding or fasting. Inflammation markers are present in adipose, or fat, tissue, where it plays a role in influencing blood glucose, which can result in metabolic diseases such as type 2 diabetes. In children, inflammation due to increased weight gain can occur at any period of development and may affect numerous organ systems. There is increasing evidence that weight reduction in children with obesity can lead to normalized levels of inflammation and improved metabolic function (Singer & Lumeng, 2017; Verbiest et al., 2021).

There is a limited body of research demonstrating that inflammation is associated with psychological factors, such as emotional eating, and that some psychological factors may influence changes in inflammation after youth participate in lifestyle interventions (Verbiest et al., 2021). Additional research is needed to confirm these findings. Nevertheless, extant evidence regarding potential interactions among biological mechanisms, psychological mechanisms, and obesity provides important insights regarding onset and maintenance of excess weight in children and adolescents. The concept of the *metabolic set point*, or *the set-point model*, may also be implicated in difficulties associated with weight loss. According to Hall and Guo (2017), energy intake and expenditure are interdependent and dynamically influenced by each other as well as by body weight. In fact, attempts to change energy balance may actually lead to physiological changes (e.g., increased appetite, suppressed energy expenditure from physical activity) that make initial weight loss and maintenance of weight loss more difficult to achieve.

Sleep deficits have also been recognized as a potential factor that is associated with increased obesity risk. The *circadian cycle* or *circadian rhythm* is a biological system that regulates physiology and metabolism through a 24-hour cycle and behaviors such as sleeping and eating (Kawai, 2022). This system can be disrupted by environmental factors, such as food availability, which can lead to metabolic complications, including obesity and impaired metabolic function. Specific disruptions attributed to sleep and weight in children include screen time before bedtime, a short sleep duration, waking up early for school, skipping breakfast, and consuming a high-fat diet. Thus, sleep deficits are another example of biological and medical factors that interact with environmental factors to influence obesity development and maintenance.

Other medical and biological factors, such as delayed feelings of fullness, hyperreactivity to environmental food cues, heightened hunger response, taking drugs that promote weight gain (e.g., steroids and psychotropic medications), and smoking cessation may also be important contributors to weight gain in adolescents and critical for clinicians to assess in determining the potential etiology and maintenance of weight gain.

MATERNAL AND DEVELOPMENTAL FACTORS

Maternal and developmental factors are recognized as important factors associated with weight gain in childhood and later the development of obesity. Maternal weight gain during pregnancy is one specific factor that has been studied. One study of more than 16,000 mothers and infants in China found that excessive weight gain early in pregnancy (e.g., first trimester weight gain in excess of medical recommendations) increased the risk of infants being born large for gestational age (Broskey et al., 2017), which is then linked to increased risk of childhood and adult obesity. Maternal gestational diabetes has also been linked to increased risk of infants being large for gestational age, childhood obesity, and development of type 2 diabetes and related glucose intolerance in childhood and adulthood (J. N. Davis et al., 2013). In the United States, prevalence rates of infants considered large for gestational age at birth are about 10% (Viswanathan et al., 2022), with women of color being more likely to give birth to a larger infant compared with non-Hispanic White women (Tutlam et al., 2017). However, breastfeeding appears to be a protective factor and may offset the impact of gestational diabetes in utero. In general, breastfeeding has been recognized as important for promoting healthy immunity development and growth in infants. The American Academy of Pediatrics recommends exclusive breastfeeding for 6 months and continuation until 1 year or longer (Section on Breastfeeding et al., 2012). Gunderson and colleagues (2018) found that, in mothers with gestational diabetes, infants who were formula fed compared with those who were primarily breast fed gained weight at a quicker rate and at earlier ages. Accelerated weight gain in infancy then increases risks for early childhood obesity (Viswanathan et al., 2022). Thus, the prenatal environment and early feeding factors appear to interact to influence later obesity and type 2 diabetes risk.

Infants born small for gestational age, defined as having a birth weight <10th percentile for gestational age (Schlaudecker et al., 2017), are also at increased risk of developing obesity later in life. Prevalence rates of small-for-gestational-age births in the United States and other developed countries are estimated to be about 11%, but in low-income and developing countries the rates are much higher (Osuchukwu & Reed, 2022). Genetic and gestational environmental factors, such as maternal nutrition and nicotine, alcohol, and drug use, have been identified as affecting fetal growth because of their impact on hormones, insulin, and growth factors, which lead to increased weight gain and eventually to the development of overweight and obesity (Nam & Lee, 2018).

Structural racism also affects maternal health before, during, and after pregnancy. Research has found that structural racism is associated with delayed prenatal care in Black women and other women of color, which raises risks for preterm birth and places infants at increased risk of being both large for gestational age and small for gestational age (Mackey et al., 2022). Racism has also been found to be associated with reduced rates of breastfeeding in Black women. Maternal factors, and their intersectionality with social determinants of health and health equity, are important considerations in understanding the etiology of pediatric obesity.

ENVIRONMENTAL FACTORS

There is evidence that environmental factors, such as the geographic characteristics of communities in which adults and children live and exposure to various environmental factors, may be associated with weight gain. Community characteristics, such as levels of urbanicity or rurality, may increase risk for developing obesity and other related comorbidities (Pirgon & Aslan, 2015). In the United States and other westernized countries, rapid urbanization has historically been identified as changing dietary and physical activity patterns that increase risks for developing obesity by limiting access to healthy foods, increasing access to unhealthy foods, and increasing engagement in sedentary behavior (Pirgon & Aslan, 2015). However, in residential areas increased walkability has been identified as a protective factor against developing obesity in children (Jia et al., 2019).

Rural communities are typically considered medically underresourced because of a lack of access to primary care and other medical providers (Agency for Healthcare Research and Quality, 2017), which may limit access to preventative services, such as evidence-based obesity prevention, assessment, and treatment (Barlow & The Expert Committee, 2007; Hampl et al., 2023b). These communities may also be affected by limited environmental infrastructure to support engagement in specific healthy lifestyle behaviors, such as consistent access to fresh fruits and vegetables and access to spaces that promote physical activity (e.g., parks, gyms, recreational spaces). Other potential issues related to rurality and obesity may include transportation distance and time; low socioeconomic status; and aspects of the rural culture, such as family structure, food environment, and access to safe outdoor activities, which influence eating and physical activity behaviors (C. S. Lim & Janicke, 2013).

Some rural and urban areas have been identified previously as *food deserts* because of limited access to grocery stores or other places to obtain fresh fruits and vegetables. However, recently these areas have been more accurately identified as *food swamps* given their lack of access to healthy foods but abundant access to unhealthy foods, such as fast food (Elbel et al., 2020); convenience stores (Xin et al., 2021); and take-out restaurants serving high-calorie, high-fat foods (M. Goodman et al., 2020). Previous research has demonstrated associations between increased risk for obesity for people living in communities characterized as food swamps (Cooksey-Stowers et al., 2017). Thus, the types of foods that are accessible in the community can contribute to the development and maintenance of pediatric obesity.

According to the obesogen hypothesis, exposure to environmental and chemical toxins may promote obesity (Heindel & Blumberg, 2019). Chemicals in the environment, which can be present in soil, food, and air, have been proposed to disrupt aspects of the endocrine system during development and influence obesity development later in life. Possible areas of impact include acting directly on cells, changing basal metabolic rate, and affecting metabolism, all of which influence the development of adipose tissue, food intake, and metabolism. Individuals may be exposed to chemical toxins through pesticides, insecticides, fungicides, fertilizers, and soil conditioners. However, research in this area is limited. Further multifactorial and longitudinal research is needed to confirm previous findings and increase understanding regarding potential impacts related to multiple chemical exposures and the potential cellular and metabolic mechanisms influenced by these chemicals, as well as identifying developmental periods sensitive to specific environmental and chemical exposures.

Other environmental factors, previously identified, are exposure to pervasive food advertising, such as for high-fat, high-sugar foods and drinks (e.g., sodas, cereal, fast food) and economic factors such as the market economy, food surplus, and westernization of food choices (e.g., fast food restaurants). Binks (2016) provided a review of the multifaceted role of the food industry specific to obesity prevention.

COGNITIVE FACTORS

Cognitive factors have also been recognized as impacting the etiology of obesity. Gunstad and colleagues (2020) proposed that neural responses to food are moderated by cognitive factors that are associated with overeating and subsequent weight gain. The influence of specific cognitive factors— attentional bias, delay discounting, and episodic memory—is supported by a growing body of research in laboratory and real-world settings demonstrating their associations with obesity development and maintenance.

First, *attentional bias* has been defined as an unconscious cognitive process that causes a person to pay attention to one type of stimuli, such as food, over another, such as non-food, because of motivational factors (Gunstad et al., 2020). Associations between attentional bias and binge eating behavior have been found, and an increased activation of brain regions associated with reward and attention has been noted in individuals with obesity. *Delay discounting* is described as an inability to delay gratification, specifically, our tendency to devalue a reward when the receipt is postponed (Gunstad et al., 2020). Poor delay discounting has been linked to increased weight status and is thought to contribute to obesity through an increased preference for high-fat, high-sugar foods, eating larger amounts of food, and eating when not hungry, as well as purchasing less healthy foods, reduced physical activity, and a decreased response to weight loss treatments. Previous research has also found that poor self-regulation skills early in childhood predict the development of obesity in later childhood (Graziano et al., 2010, 2013). Memory is an additional cognitive factor thought to influence eating and food choices through decision-making abilities. Deficits in *episodic memory*, which is the recollection of every day events and personal experiences (Tulving, 2002), has been linked to decreased adherence to weight loss treatment recommendations (Gunstad et al., 2020). Overall, the research that has examined these cognitive factors has primarily focused on adults; thus, knowledge about their potential role in pediatric obesity is limited. However, Gunstad et al. (2020) posited that these cognitive factors provide links between intentions and behaviors and are essential components of obesity prevention and effective weight management. Taken together, these findings suggest that psychologists and other health care providers working with patients and families should consider these cognitive factors when developing pediatric obesity prevention and treatment strategies.

CAREGIVER FACTORS

Caregivers are also important to consider, given both the genetic and environmental links between youth and caregiver weight status. Caregivers have been identified as important models of lifestyle behaviors—specifically, eating and physical activity—for youth. Caregivers influence child eating behaviors in a variety of ways, such as actively making food choices for the family, serving as models for dietary choices and patterns, and using feeding practices to reinforce the development of eating patterns and behaviors they feel are appropriate and, conversely, punishing or ignoring eating patterns and behaviors they feel are not appropriate (Birch et al., 2007). Parenting styles have also been associated with feeding and eating behaviors; specifically, an *authoritarian parenting style*, which is characterized by pressure to eat, restrictive feeding, and low responsiveness to the child's needs, are thought to promote overeating, food rejection, picky eating, and an increased risk for becoming overweight (Birch et al., 2007; S. O. Hughes et al., 2005), compared with the *authoritative parenting style*, which is characterized by parental support and high responsiveness to the child's needs and eating cues and has been found to promote healthier child eating behaviors (Birch et al., 2007; Rhee et al., 2006).

Research also suggests that caregivers play a role in youth engagement in physical activity. Caregiver modeling of physical activity is positively associated with increased youth physical activity (Pugliese & Tinsley, 2007). However, research indicates that some parenting styles are associated with levels of youth physical activity (Hennessy et al., 2010; Janssen, 2015), and caregiver support has been identified as an important factor that affects physical activity, especially for children to engage in physical activities of moderate to vigorous intensity (Langer et al., 2014; Trost et al., 2003). For example, caregivers sign children up for extracurricular activities, such as for team and individual sports, as well as other activities, which may range from active to sedentary. Caregivers' own perceptions, experiences, knowledge, and attitudes regarding structured and unstructured physical activities, as well as perceptions of safety in the community for children to engage in physical activity, and economic resources that support engagement in exercise, are important factors regarding youth engagement in physical activity.

FAMILY AND SOCIAL FACTORS

Adversity and dysfunction in the social environment, including parental and family relationships, during infancy and early childhood have been recognized as a social determinant of health for a variety of physical and mental health outcomes. These have also been specifically identified as risk factors for weight gain and the development of obesity in youth. In addition to the parent, family, and social factors included in The Obesity Society (2015) infographic (Figure 4.1) the *family ecological model*, which combines ecological and family systems theories, accounts for contextual and family factors that affect parenting specific to healthy lifestyle behaviors (Davison et al., 2013). The model posits that family ecology, consisting of family history and structure, child-specific characteristics, organizational factors, community factors, and media and policy factors, influences family knowledge and social norms, as well as social disparities and chronic stress, which then affect parenting behaviors and practices and children's cognitions and behaviors that lead to caregiver and child health outcomes specific to obesity and associated medical conditions (see Figure 4.2).

Limited financial resources associated with poverty and low socioeconomic status have been deemed critical risk factors for pediatric obesity via indirect promotion of unhealthy lifestyle choices, stress, and family dysfunction (Hemmingsson, 2018). In terms of indirectly promoting unhealthy eating, some researchers have proposed that families with low financial resources and caregivers with less education may be more susceptible to pervasive unhealthy food advertising (Hemmingsson, 2018). Limited access to economic resources and education about healthy lifestyle behaviors may also result in low knowledge and prioritization of healthy lifestyle behaviors by caregivers and children. For example, living in a crime-prone area may limit engagement in outdoor physical activity and increase sedentary behavior because of safety concerns (The Obesity Society, 2015). In addition, lack of access to health care is associated with lower economic resources. Limited access to health care results in inadequate nutritional support from dietitians and a lack of health care provider support or knowledge of obesity prevention and treatment efforts. Living in poverty or having limited access to resources also causes increased stress on caregivers. Sources of stress may include economic and employment pressure, housing instability, food insecurity, limited social support, disruption of family routines and relationships, transportation and child care issues, and other competing priorities (Davison et al., 2013). Other sources of stress experienced by caregivers who are from racial/ethnic minority groups include discrimination; structural racism in education, occupation and housing; food availability and marketing; physical activity resources; availability of health care settings; and health disparities (Mackey et al., 2022). Chronic stress in caregivers is associated with neglect, relationship discord, and mental health problems, all of which can result in a harsh and insecure social environment during critical periods of development for infants and young children (Hemmingsson, 2018). Previous research has linked these factors to later weight gain and obesity development.

Other social factors linked to the development of obesity are weight bias and stigma (Puhl et al., 2020; Chapter 3, this volume), which can occur in a variety of settings, such as school, family, and health care settings. Children with obesity are also at significantly increased risk for experiencing teasing, bullying, and peer victimization as a result of their body size and shape

FIGURE 4.2. The Revised Family Ecological Model

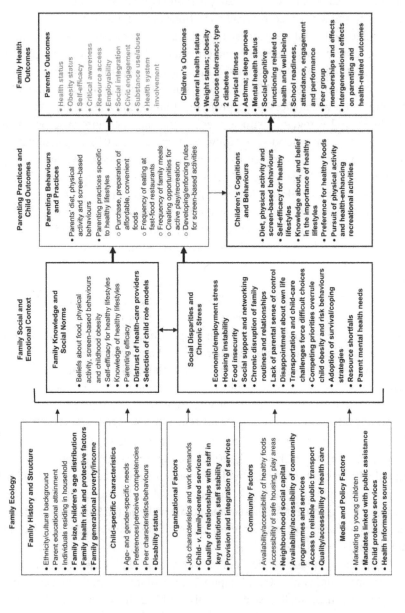

Note. From "Reframing Family-Centred Obesity Prevention Using the Family Ecological Model," by K. K. Davison, J. M. Jurkowski, and H. A. Lawson, 2013, *Public Health Nutrition, 16*(10), p. 1867 (https://doi.org/10.1017/S1368980012004533). Reprinted with permission.

(Puhl et al., 2017). These negative experiences may lead to limited engagement in physical activity and healthy eating behaviors or, conversely, result in increased engagement in unhealthy lifestyle behaviors, which then lead to weight gain, throughout childhood, adolescence, and adulthood.

PSYCHOLOGICAL FACTORS

The Obesity Society (2015) infographic includes specific psychological factors, which are also important to consider as potential contributors to energy storage or increased weight. These specific psychological factors include disordered eating (e.g., nighttime eating, binge eating, food addiction), emotional coping, self-regulatory and coping deficits (e.g., emotional eating), trauma history, mood disturbance (e.g., depression, anxiety, bipolar disorder), developmental disabilities, social anxiety, stress, and weight cycling (also referred to as *yo-yo dieting*). We review these factors in more detail in Part III of this book, when we discuss approaches to pediatric obesity prevention and treatment that specifically take these psychological factors and symptoms into account.

LIFESTYLE BEHAVIORS

Dietary intake and physical activity are the primary lifestyle behaviors that have been studied to address the development and maintenance of pediatric obesity, mostly because effective treatments targeting other etiology factors are limited. This has resulted in decades of targeting lifestyle behaviors as they pertain to prevention and treatment strategies to address childhood obesity. Table 4.1 identifies specific lifestyle behaviors to target that are based on expert treatment recommendations for the prevention and treatment of pediatric obesity (Barlow & The Expert Committee, 2007).

CONCLUSION

As reviewed, many factors contribute to the development and maintenance of obesity in youth. Obesity is a complex, multifactorial chronic medical condition (Heindel & Blumberg, 2019); however, there are limited effective treatments currently available that directly address genetic, biological, societal, and other factors. Despite specific causes or factors, and the intersection of various etiologies, it is important for psychologists and other mental health

TABLE 4.1. Recommendations for Specific Lifestyle Behaviors to Target Specific Lifestyle Behaviors to Prevention and Treatment of Pediatric Obesity

Recommendations	Prevention	Stage 1: Prevention Plus	Stage 2: Structured Weight Management	Stage 3: Comprehensive Interdisciplinary Intervention	Stage 4: Tertiary Care Intervention
Recommended ages	Applicable to all children starting at birth	Youth 2–19 years with BMI ≥85th percentile with health risks	After 3–6 months of Prevention Plus and no improvement	Youth 6+ years with BMI ≥95th percentile (or BMI 85th–94th percentile with health risks)	Youth 11+ years old with BMI ≥95th percentile with comorbidities or BMI ≥99th percentile
Target behaviors	• Limit sugar sweetened beverages • Consume fruits and vegetables (consistent with USDA recommendations) • Decrease screen time and sedentary behavior • Eat breakfast daily • Limit eating out • Have family meals • Decrease portion sizes • Diet high in calcium and fiber and balanced fat, carbs, and protein • Exclusive breast feeding for 6 months and then to 12 months or longer • Moderate to vigorous physical activity for at least 1 hour/day • Limit high-calorie foods	• 5+ fruits and vegetables/day • Minimize sugar-sweetened beverages • Decrease screen time to <2 hours/day • 1+ hour of physical activity each day • Prepare meals at home • Family meals at table 5–6 times a week • Eat a healthy breakfast each day • Involve the whole family • Allow child to self-regulate meals and avoid overly restrictive feeding • Tailor recommendations to family and cultural values	• Target behaviors in Prevention Plus and: – Planned diet or daily eating plan with balanced nutrients – Structured eating plan (3 meals & 1–2 snacks, no caloric beverages) – Further reduce screen time and sedentary behavior to <1 hour/day – Planned supervised 1+ hour of physical activity each day – Monitor behaviors with logs – Plan reinforcement for achieving targeted goals	• Behavior modification program • Negative energy balance • Intensive parent participation (somewhat less in youth age 13+) • Focus on home environment • Systematic evaluations of health and weight status and dietary intake and physical activity • Interdisciplinary team • Frequent visits (ideally weekly for 8–12 weeks) • Group sessions	• Restrictive diet • FDA-approved medications • Weight control surgery

| Recommended setting | • Primary care | • Primary care | • Primary care with health care providers (e.g., dietitian, clinician) trained in motivational interviewing and behavioral strategies (e.g., monitoring, reinforcement) | • Established pediatric weight management program (if available)
• Commercial weight management program (after being screened by primary care for appropriateness) | • Established pediatric weight management program | • Established pediatric weight management program |

Note. This table was created on the basis of information presented in Barlow and The Expert Committee (2007). BMI = body mass index; USDA = U.S. Department of Agriculture; FDA = U.S. Food and Drug Administration providers working to prevent and treat childhood obesity to ensure interventions are tailored to the child and family (e.g., biological, social, psychological) and the community (e.g., context) in which they live and that they account for the various social determinants of health that are recognized risk factors for obesity in youth (Hampl et al., 2023a).

KEY POINTS

- The factors leading to the development and intractability of obesity are numerous.
- More research is needed to develop and examine prevention and treatment strategies that target intersecting etiologies, including social determinants of health and structural racism.

THINKING OUTSIDE THE BOX

How do weight stigma and structural racism intersect in health care settings?

PART II

PREVENTION AND TREATMENT OF PEDIATRIC OBESITY

In Part II, we review general psychological techniques that have been applied to the prevention and treatment of pediatric obesity and provide example materials for practitioners to consider using. We also discuss prevention and treatment approaches in various contexts, such as school settings and retail and immersion programs. The use of medications and surgery for the treatment of pediatric obesity is reviewed, as are psychological considerations mental health care providers should consider when implementing these treatment approaches with youth with obesity and their families.

5 PSYCHOLOGICAL TECHNIQUES IN THE PREVENTION AND TREATMENT OF PEDIATRIC OBESITY

There are numerous psychological techniques that can be implemented in the prevention and treatment of pediatric obesity. Much of the previous research that has examined the efficacy and effectiveness of pediatric obesity prevention and treatments implemented in multicomponent lifestyle treatment programs, in which multiple health behaviors are targeted and health behavior change is encouraged through the use of a variety of behavioral, cognitive, and parenting strategies. Thus, in general, the research is not clear with regard to which components are the most important or most effective and which strategies work the best for some families or youth and not others. In this chapter, we review and discuss general psychological strategies that can assist in the treatment of pediatric obesity, and later in the book (Part III) we review other strategies to address specific developmental and psychological concerns experienced by pediatric patients with overweight and obesity.

https://doi.org/10.1037/0000401-005
Psychological Approaches to the Treatment of Pediatric Obesity, by C. S. Lim and E. T. Burton

MOTIVATIONAL INTERVIEWING

Motivational interviewing is a psychological technique that was initially developed for therapists working with individuals with substance use disorders (Rollnick et al., 2008). However, in the past few decades it has been implemented with a variety of adult and child/pediatric populations. Motivational interviewing has been found to be effective at improving a variety of health behaviors, including substance use, smoking cessation, HIV risk, hemoglobin A1c values, treatment compliance, and lifestyle behaviors (dietary intake and physical activity; Gourlan et al., 2013; Martins & McNeil, 2009; Resnicow et al., 2006). Motivational interviewing has been defined as a style of helping individuals identify their own interests and motivations to change their behavior, leading to health improvements (Rollnick et al., 2008). Motivational interviewing is distinct from traditional health and mental health care because it is more collaborative, evocative, and autonomous—health behaviors and strategies to change those behaviors are identified by both the patient and the provider, clients identify their own motivation and resources to change, and the client chooses ultimately whether or not to change their behavior (Rollnick et al., 2008). In 2007, when the American Academy of Pediatrics released their expert treatment recommendations for the prevention, assessment, and treatment of pediatric obesity, motivational interviewing was a key patient-centered counseling technique identified as being important for pediatricians and interdisciplinary treatment team members, such as psychologists, to help facilitate lifestyle behavior change in children and their families (Barlow & The Expert Committee, 2007). In the updated American Academy of Pediatrics clinical practice guidelines for the treatment of youth with obesity, motivational interviewing is specifically referred to in a key action statement to be used by pediatricians and other primary health care providers to engage youth and their families when treating overweight and obesity (Hampl et al., 2023a). In Table 5.1 we provide specific aspects and components of motivational interviewing that could apply to the treatment of pediatric obesity, as well as specific example statements and questions that are consistent with the intention and principles of motivational interviewing for health behavior change. Some key features of motivational interviewing are that it can be used to identify youth and family reasons for weight management, to modify multiple lifestyle behaviors, and it can be used in conjunction with the other treatment strategies discussed throughout this book.

TABLE 5.1. Applying Brief Motivational Interviewing to Pediatric Obesity Prevention and Treatment

Important components of brief motivational interviewing for pediatric obesity
Nondirective, collaborative approach
• Use open-ended questions (aim for about 70%)
• Reflective listening
• Comparison of current health behaviors and values (limit judgment by normalizing challenges)
• Implement problem solving to address potential barriers
• Develop realistic and gradual goals
• Focus on successes (no matter how small!)
Example use of motivational interviewing in pediatric obesity treatment
Assess weight status and healthy lifestyle behaviors
• *Example:* How many (8-oz) cups of sweet beverages (e.g., sweet tea, soda, fruit drinks [not 100% juice], Gatorade) does your child currently drink each day?
Identify target behaviors
• *Example:* What do you think you and your child could change in relation to your family's activity level?
Assess motivation and confidence
• *Example:* On a scale of 0 to 10, with 10 being very important, how important is it for you to reduce the amount of fast food your child eats?
• *Example:* On a scale of 0 to 10, with 10 being very confident, how confident are you that you will try at least one new vegetable this week?
Summarize possible changes
• *Example:* How can you fit physical activity into your family's daily routine?
Schedule a follow-up visit
• *Example:* Let's schedule a follow-up visit to see how things are going. When would you like to come back so we can check in about your family's progress with these goals?

Note. This table was developed on the basis of information presented in Barlow and The Expert Committee (2007) and Rollnick et al. (2008).

MONITORING LIFESTYLE BEHAVIORS

Decades of research and clinical practice with adults enrolled in weight management programs have emphasized the importance of self-monitoring lifestyle behaviors, such as eating and physical activity. In addition, the American Psychological Association (APA; 2013) identified that one role psychologists can play in weight management is to teach self-monitoring skills. Self-monitoring can be helpful for a variety of reasons, such as increasing awareness of lifestyle behaviors, enhancing feelings of control over eating and physical activity behaviors, identifying problematic habits and thinking patterns related to food and physical activity, helping individuals make changes, and identifying areas of positive change (Cooper et al., 2003). In fact, recent research with adults suggests that greater adherence to recommended self-monitoring specific to dietary intake, physical activity, and weight resulted in increased weight loss (S. P. Goldstein et al., 2019). Research focused on monitoring in children and caregivers participating in pediatric weight management trials have revealed similar results. Germann and colleagues (2007) found that children who self-monitored their eating and physical activity for most days lost more weight than those who were less consistent with monitoring lifestyle behaviors. Children whose caregiver self-monitored were more likely to also self-monitor and lose weight during the initial 3 months of treatment. In addition to eating behaviors and engagement in physical activity, monitoring can be used to focus on other health behaviors, such as sleep and medication use, as well as to keep track of emotions, thoughts, and behaviors that may be important to incorporate into weight management treatment. An example pencil-and-paper monitoring form that can be used by children and families to monitor eating and physical activity behaviors is depicted in Figure 5.1.

Increased access to technology, via smartphones, tablets, smartwatches, pedometers, and other app- and sensor-based activity trackers, has led to additional electronic health (eHealth) and mobile health (mHealth) options for monitoring healthy lifestyle behaviors. In general, mobile health technologies have been found to be user friendly, acceptable, and feasible to implement in pediatric weight management treatments (Turner et al., 2015). Meta analyses indicated that mobile technologies focused on self-monitoring had a significant and small effect on weight status in youth (Darling & Sato, 2017). However, the impacts of these technologies on eating behaviors and physical activity have revealed very small to inconclusive significant effect sizes, respectively (Darling & Sato, 2017). Psychologists and other mental health providers can help provide education to youth and their families regarding the importance of self-monitoring, identify important lifestyle behaviors to target, suggest ways to implement self-monitoring in their everyday lives, identify the type of monitoring (e.g., pencil and paper, electronic) that is most feasible for the child and caregiver, and problem-solve with families when issues may arise related to monitoring lifestyle behaviors.

GOAL SETTING

In the treatment of pediatric obesity, psychologists and other mental health care providers collaborate with families to improve weight management through behavior change. In treatment settings, families may seek services

FIGURE 5.1. Example Daily Healthy Lifestyle Monitoring Log

Day of the Week: _____   Date: _____

Eating/drinking		
Time	**Specific food/drink**	**How much/many?**
BREAKFAST		
LUNCH		
DINNER		
SNACKS		
Physical activity		

TOTAL STEPS	

"Non-step" activities (i.e., bike, swimming)	How long?

and have a specific goal in mind related to weight loss. However, these identified goals often are unattainable or unrealistic and may actually be harmful (e.g., significant weight loss in short period of time). One important way to change behavior is through modifying lifestyle habits gradually. Psychologists and other mental health care providers can play an important role in helping families set realistic and obtainable goals related to specific healthy lifestyle behaviors (as opposed to a specific weight or health outcome). Ross and colleagues (2010) recommended using the acronym SMART, which refers to setting and identifying goals that are Specific, Measurable, Achievable, Realistic, and Timely. Education regarding each component of SMART goal setting is provided to pediatric patients and their caregivers, and then a specific lifestyle behavior is identified and targeted. At future sessions or clinic visits, the goal and plan to achieve that goal are reviewed and modified on the basis of barriers or successes. Other acronyms have also been used to teach goal setting, such as STAR (Specific, Testable, Attainable, and Relevant; Learning Assistance Centre, University of Manitoba, 2023). An example SMART problem-solving worksheet implemented in outpatient pediatric obesity medical clinic settings is presented in Figure 5.2.

An additional strategy specific to goal setting is the use of *guided goal setting*. Guided goal setting has been characterized as the psychologist or mental health provider developing a list of multiple potential goals and the youth and/or caregiver choosing one goal to work on (Shilts et al., 2004). Shilts and colleagues (2018) examined an obesity prevention program for caregivers with young children that incorporated this specific goal-setting technique. In this 6-week program, caregivers first completed an assessment focused on nutrition, physical activity, and feeding behaviors associated with pediatric obesity and then were given positive feedback regarding one area and given suggestions about two areas for improvement. Caregivers then selected one of these areas as a primary goal and selected an additional minor goal from a predetermined list. In follow-up sessions, caregivers were given options to continue with the same goal, modify the goal, select a goal from the guided list, or create a new goal. At the end of the program, quantitative results revealed that caregivers reported eating out less often and served fewer sugar-sweetened beverages and unhealthy snacks. Qualitatively, caregivers indicated that personalizing goals was the most useful part of the prevention program. Providing youth and their caregivers with a predetermined set of healthy lifestyle goals may help facilitate the goal-setting process, especially in settings where time spent with individual families may be limited or impractical. This approach would also demonstrate that other families have similar difficulties with specific healthy lifestyle behaviors.

FIGURE 5.2. Example SMART Goals Worksheet

SETTING SMART GOALS

- **S = Specific:** Use specific rather than general language. Describe exactly what, who, where, and when. Clearly state the issue, the target behavior, who will be involved, and the time and place it will occur.
- **M = Measurable:** Be clear in the objective about what will be changed and by how much. State how much? Or how many? Include days, times, and amounts! Setting this clearly at the start makes it easier to evaluate.
- **A = Achievable:** Be realistic about what can be achieved in terms of the scale/scope of what is being done, the time and resources available. Is there anything that you need before you can work on your goal? What barriers do you foresee that might interfere with your ability to achieve your goal?
- **R = Realistic:** Objectives need to relate to and be relevant to the goals. Remember, objectives are the building blocks/steps toward meeting the goals.
- **T = Time-based:** Be clear about the time frame in which the behavior changes will take place. Set specific start and end dates or timeframes.

Example SMART Goal: I will replace potato chips with grapes at lunch. I will serve Johnny ½ cup of grapes every day at lunch beginning tomorrow and until Friday. First, I will stop and buy a bag of grapes on my way home from clinic tonight. Then, when I get home, I will throw away or donate all the potato chips in our house.

SMART Goal #1:_____

_____

_____

SMART Goal #2:_____

_____

_____

PROBLEM SOLVING

When discussing goals with children and families, it is also important to assess expected barriers to changing healthy lifestyle behaviors. Psychologists and other mental health care providers may consider integrating various problem-solving strategies with families in pediatric obesity prevention and treatment settings. The structure of problem solving can vary, and numerous versions of problem solving have been implemented in family therapy and treatment programs for caregivers of children with chronic medical conditions. *Behavioral family systems therapy* incorporates principles of behavioral and family systems theory, and problem solving is included as a component (Quittner et al., 2000). It has been implemented with various pediatric populations, such as individuals with type 1 diabetes (H. Wang et al., 2021), asthma (Carr, 2019), and cystic fibrosis (Quittner et al., 2000), to improve medication adherence.

Some psychological treatments have been developed to specifically target problem solving skills. For example, *problem-solving skills training* was initially developed for caregivers of children diagnosed with cancer and is a short-term (e.g., eight sessions) treatment designed to teach skills that involve effective problem solving, including skills that address various problems faced by caregivers (APA, 2011; Sahler et al., 2013). Problem-solving skills training has since been modified and implemented in various child clinical and pediatric populations, such as autism (Nguyen et al., 2016), asthma (Seid et al., 2010), and chronic pain (Palermo et al., 2014).

If not incorporated as part of a specific treatment, general psychoeducation regarding problem-solving steps can be considered for the prevention and treatment of pediatric obesity. Various acronyms to help youth and families learn the steps to problem solving have been developed and implemented; one is IDEAL (Identify the problem, Define the goal, Explore possible solutions through brainstorming and evaluating options, Agree and make a plan, Look back and check progress).

Figure 5.3 is an example problem-solving worksheet providers could consider reviewing and implementing with children and families in various pediatric obesity treatment settings.

STIMULUS CONTROL

An additional concept that has been recognized as important for the treatment of pediatric obesity is stimulus control. In weight management programs, stimulus control focuses on changing the environment to promote positive health behaviors (Dalton & Kitzmann, 2012). The focus is specific to eating

FIGURE 5.3. Example IDEAL Problem-Solving Worksheet

IDEAL Problem-Solving Worksheet

I – Identify the problem: _____

D – Define the goal: _____

_____

E – Explore possible solutions:

Possible solutions	Rating (+ or −)
1)	
2)	
3)	
4)	
5)	

A – Agree and make a plan:

Solution:_____

Responsibilities for each family member (list name and responsibilities):

_____

Signatures:

_____ Date: _____

_____ Date: _____

L – Look back and check progress

and involves recognizing eating cues and implementing specific cues only during meals and snacks, as well as removing unhealthy foods from the home and replacing them with healthy food choices (Carr, 2019). In this approach, the environment is modified by making the healthy choice the easier option for the child and family (Bejarano et al., 2019). Scheduled family mealtimes and eating only at a table, with electronic screens off, are examples of food cues that may be important for psychologists and other mental health care providers to consider discussing with children and caregivers. Stimulus control has also been implemented to increase physical activity and decrease sedentary behavior; specifically, changes to the environment are made to limit sedentary behavior, including engaging with electronic screen only during specified times and disconnecting from screens at other times (Epstein et al., 2004).

MINDFUL EATING

Mindful eating is based on mindfulness, which is a component of various empirically supported psychological treatments. In general, mindfulness is thought to consist of attention to the immediate experience, increased recognition of the present moment, and interpreting the present moment with curiosity, acceptance, and openness (Bishop et al., 2004). In adults, mindfulness-based therapeutic approaches are effective treatments for anxiety, depression, and stress (Khoury et al., 2013) and have demonstrated promising effects at reducing psychological symptoms in youth (Zoogman et al., 2015). The growing body of research evidence regarding the effectiveness of mindfulness has led to the implementation of the approach with individuals who have chronic medical conditions.

Mindful eating has been incorporated into obesity treatments for adults and has been described as involving encouraging individuals to pay attention to various sensations when they are eating, including savoring each bite and noticing specific aspects of food, such as tastes and textures (Cooper et al., 2003). There is research support that mindfulness improves eating behaviors and weight status, as well as psychological symptoms such as depression and anxiety, in adults with overweight and obesity (Rogers et al., 2017). A more recent meta-analysis that included only randomized controlled trials comparing mindfulness approaches with control conditions had mixed findings: There were significant improvements in binge eating symptoms compared with control conditions but no significant difference in weight status in adults (Mercado et al., 2021). Mindfulness-based interventions have also been evaluated in adolescents. Shomaker and colleagues (2019) found improvements in depressive symptoms and insulin resistance in adolescents with overweight or obesity after participating in a 1-year mindfulness-based group intervention even though significant changes in weight status were not found.

In youth with overweight and obesity, mindful eating is hypothesized to lead to improved coping with distressing emotions, increased awareness of emotional and physical cues that influence eating, and compassion leading to body satisfaction and self-acceptance (Dalen et al., 2015). In addition, specific to cooking and family-based approaches, mindfulness can apply to grocery shopping, such as attention to the cost and healthfulness of food purchased; to food preparation and awareness of kitchen safety; and to food consumption, such as paying attention to serving sizes and satiety cues (Burton & Smith, 2020). Thus, mindful eating is thought to increase awareness regarding the connections among emotions, eating cues, and eating behaviors, as well as other external and internal factors.

Mindful eating has been included as the primary treatment, or part of interdisciplinary and multicomponent treatments, for pediatric overweight and obesity. For example, Kumar and colleagues (2018) conducted a pilot randomized controlled trial that compared a four-session mindful eating intervention with standard dietary counseling for adolescents with obesity. The intervention was acceptable and feasible, but no group differences in weight or health status were found. In addition, Burton and Smith (2020) developed and integrated a culturally tailored mindful eating program into family-based cooking classes for youth with overweight or obesity receiving services in their pediatric weight management clinic that primarily treated Black families living in underresourced communities. Although empirical evidence is not currently available, anecdotal results have revealed high participation and satisfaction and low attrition, suggesting that a culturally tailored mindful eating approach, when integrated with cooking classes, is an acceptable intervention for racially diverse families.

In summary, mindfulness interventions and mindful eating strategies could be important components in the prevention and treatment of pediatric obesity, can be implemented in a variety of clinical and community settings, and appear to be helpful in racially diverse families to whom psychologists and other mental health care providers may provide services. However, additional research is needed to continue examining both the efficacy and effectiveness of mindfulness approaches to both prevent and treat pediatric obesity, especially in racial and ethnically diverse and underresourced families. Figure 5.4 provides a mindful eating handout and related exercise.

FIGURE 5.4. Mindful Eating Handout and Exercise

Mindful Eating

MINDFULNESS – *WHAT Skills* and *HOW Skills* provide the basis of mindfulness and mindful eating.

WHAT Skills (help you know what to do)

- *Observe*
  - Be on the alert—notice what is going on inside (thoughts, feelings, sensations) and outside (environment, temperature) without reacting, adding anything to it, judging it, or trying to change it.
  - Allow your thoughts, feelings, and sensations to come and go, as if they are on a conveyor belt.
  - Push nothing away (no matter how uncomfortable/painful) and hold onto nothing (no matter how enjoyable/pleasant).
- *Describe*
  - Label what you have observed and notice what works.
  - Keep it simple and descriptive:
    - For example: "I feel sad" or "My face feels hot."
  - Stick with just the facts—describe only what you observe, without interpretations:
    - Instead of "That person has an attitude," describe that person, such as "rolling their eyes, speaking with a loud voice," and so on.
- *Participate*
  - Be here now—try not to worry about the past or the future; focus on the present.
  - Fully experience your life without being self-conscious.
  - Be a part of what's happening without needing to love it or hate it.
  - Practice letting go of thoughts like "How am I doing" or "How do I look?"

HOW Skills (help you know how to do it)

- *Do not judge*
  - Notice what is going on without labeling as good or bad.
  - Acknowledge how things affect you, but don't judge it:
    - For example, replace "You are a jerk" with "I feel mad when you walk away when we are talking."
  - Do not judge your judging:
    - You cannot go through life without making judgments; the goal is to catch your judgments so you have more control over your emotions.
- *Stay focused*
  - Do one thing at a time (this is the opposite of multitasking).
  - Give your full attention to whatever you are doing.
  - Concentrate and let go of distractions:
    - For example, choose to listen to music without checking text messages, Facebook, X, TikTok, etc.

FIGURE 5.4. Mindful Eating Handout and Exercise (*Continued*)

- *Do what works*
  - ○ Be productive and do what you need to do to work toward your goals.
  - ○ It is okay to make mistakes—just be sure to learn from them.
  - ○ Focus on what works—do not get caught up in what is right or wrong, fair or unfair.
  - ○ Let go of negative feelings that can hurt (e.g., extreme anger, revenge) and make things worse.
  - ○ Act as skillfully as you can.

MINDFUL EATING: By eating mindfully, we slow down the eating process and can pay more attention to the feeling of fullness.

This consists of

- Eating with awareness.
- Paying attention to your experiences of eating.
- Being in control of your experience of eating rather than letting your eating be in control of you.

Use all 3 **WHAT Skills** when eating:

- *Observe*—How does the food look, smell, taste, feel, etc., in your mouth?
- *Describe*—Focus on the vibrant color, sweet smell, tart taste, smooth texture, etc.
- *Participate*—Pay attention to the experience of eating.

Example Mindful Eating Activity:

Provide individual with an orange. Read the following instructions:

- "Admire the color, shape, and texture of the fruit. Oranges grow on trees in warm climates. Close your eyes and imagine where your orange grew. Can you feel the warm sun? Can you smell the blossoms? Can you see the fruit on the trees?"
- "Open your eyes and smell the orange. Place the orange on a napkin or piece of paper towel. Roll the orange firmly on the table to release the orange essence. Pick up the orange again and smell the essence."
- "Begin to peel the skin off the orange. Notice changes in smells, textures, and appearance. Take time to smell the orange again. Does it smell stronger? Sweeter? Peel the fruit slowly, taking time to enjoy the aroma, texture, and color."
- "Separate the segments of the orange. Examine their inner structure – hundreds of tiny juice-filled sacs. Place a segment in your mouth, close your eyes, and bite down. Pay attention to how the juice bursts into your mouth and fills it with orange flavor. Chew slowly and experience the texture of the membrane."
- "Continue eating your orange, and as you chew slowly, pretend this is the last orange on earth. It's all yours!"

Reflect and discuss the experience.

- "How was this different from your general orange-eating experiences?"
- "More intense? Frustrating? More pleasurable?"
- "Were you more aware of your emotions during the exercise?"
- "Would this change your future experience of eating oranges? Why?"

Note. This figure was developed on the basis of information presented in Pluhar et al. (2018), Linehan (1993a), and Rathus and Miller (2014).

PARENTING STRATEGIES

Psychologists have developed various parenting programs with many different names (e.g., parent management training [PMT], parent–child interaction therapy [PCIT]) that teach caregivers skills to modify problematic child behaviors. Most often, these programs target families who have a child with attention-deficit/hyperactivity disorder or oppositional defiant disorder. However, many of the same parenting strategies implemented in these programs, such as praise, reinforcement, and differential attention, have been modified and integrated into family-based interventions to address pediatric overweight and obesity. Including parent management and behavioral strategies can help caregivers learn to better manage children's reactions to changes in eating and physical activity, as well as possible noncompliance or misbehavior that might arise when changes are being implemented (Bejarano et al., 2019).

Praise

Epstein and Squires's (1988) Stoplight Diet, on which previous and current pediatric obesity treatments are often based, focuses on the importance of praise and rewards. Praise and rewards are consistent with *positive reinforcement*, or providing a stimulus that increases the chance a positive behavior will happen again. Epstein and Squires's research suggests that when caregivers use frequent praise in pediatric weight management programs children are able to change their lifestyle behaviors, lose more weight, and sustain weight loss. However, it is also important for psychologists and other mental health care providers working in pediatric obesity treatment settings to teach caregivers, and remember themselves, to provide praise—specifically, labeled praise—that is based on behavior change and not on weight loss. For example, avoid general statements like "Great job!" and provide more specific praise, such as "Great job replacing your chips with fruits and vegetables for your snacks!" In addition, the focus on specific behaviors and not weight loss is thought to prevent children from engaging in unhealthy or disordered eating behaviors in order to lose weight. Similar to the general parent management programs, in parent-focused pediatric weight management programs caregivers are usually taught the most effective ways to give praise, given opportunities to role-play and practice, and then receive coaching or feedback from program leaders when giving their child praise, to improve their specific parenting skills (Janicke et al., 2013).

Reward Systems

Token economies, or reward charts, are another parent management strategy applicable to pediatric obesity prevention and treatment. For some children, only receiving praise for changing their behavior, whether it be disruptive behavior or engaging in healthy lifestyle behaviors, is not enough to result in long-term behavior change (Barkley, 2013). They need extra support and motivation to engage in healthier lifestyle behaviors early in a pediatric obesity prevention or treatment program. The reward system should focus on specific behaviors, such as trying new fruits and vegetables or engaging in physical activity, and not weight loss. Reward systems typically involve the child earning privileges or rewards and consist of both short-term (e.g., multiple times a day, daily) and long-term rewards (e.g., weekly, monthly; Barkley, 2013; Epstein & Squires, 1988). The reward system should also be developed in a way that is consistent with eating cues and mindful eating; specifically, providers need to ensure that caregivers use nonfood rewards (e.g., stickers, tokens, points), which may be an important change for the family.

Behavioral Contracts

Behavioral contracts are another tool that has been implemented in pediatric obesity prevention and treatment programs and that may be more useful with older children and adolescents. These typically are a formal agreement between the caregiver and child that is contingent on the youth engaging in specific healthy lifestyle behaviors, such as monitoring their eating, eating specific numbers of vegetables and fruits, and engaging in a specific amount of physical activity. These contracts typically also include a combination of short-term (e.g., daily) and long-term rewards and privileges (e.g., weekly, monthly; Epstein & Squires, 1988). The key when developing contracts is that the child and caregiver are in agreement and the rewards are developmentally appropriate and individualized to the child and family. A signed contract encourages accountability and follow-through with the agreed-on conditions for the child to receive the rewards.

Differential Attention

Differential attention is traditionally used in parent management programs in combination with praise and rewards. It refers to targeting child behaviors a caregiver wants to decrease by using both ignoring, for inappropriate behavior, and positive attention, for appropriate behavior (Hembree-Kigin & McNeil,

1995). In pediatric obesity prevention and treatment programs, this is a tool caregivers are taught and encouraged to use in order to reduce child complaints or whining about healthy eating and physical activity behavior changes. For example, if the target child is complaining about having to eat a new vegetable, a caregiver would be encouraged to ignore complaints and praise other siblings and family members for trying the vegetable. In addition, as soon as the target child eats or drinks something healthy or makes a positive statement about healthy eating, the caregiver would immediately provide labeled praise.

Role of Caregivers

Depending on the age of the child, many clinicians and researchers conceptualize caregivers as agents of change in pediatric weight management (Ball et al., 2012; Bejarano et al., 2019; Epstein & Squires, 1988; Golan, 2006). This is mostly because young children have little control over what foods and drinks are brought into the home and limited influence on the physical activities that are encouraged and implemented. Caregivers also model healthy lifestyle behaviors: If children see caregivers making changes to their eating and physical activity behaviors, it will be easier for children to adopt and follow through with similar changes (Bejarano et al., 2019). There is evidence that pediatric weight management interventions that include only caregivers (as opposed to both children and caregivers, or only children) result in greater improvements in weight status for both caregivers and children (Golan, 2006); thus, treatment programs focused on childhood obesity need to consider the role of caregivers.

Cultural Considerations

When implementing parenting interventions to modify health behaviors, it is vital to consider the family culture. Taking into account various cultural influences, such as cultural beliefs, cultural traditions, and structural issues (e.g., socioeconomic status, access to resources) on caregivers, children, and families, as well as family perceptions and beliefs regarding parenting, are necessary to ensure the appropriateness and applicability of obesity treatments (N. J. Taylor et al., 2013). For example, there is some evidence that parents from diverse racial and ethnic backgrounds may use different parental feeding strategies more often compared with non-Hispanic White parents (C. S. Lim et al., 2019; Wehrly et al., 2014). Parent use of pressure or forcing a child to eat is thought to disrupt self-regulation related to eating, which can lead to weight gain and obesity (Wehrly et al., 2014). However, research is limited, and the role different parental feeding strategies may play in increased obesity risk or response to parent-focused pediatric obesity treatments is unclear. More research that examines cultural considerations in parenting and parent feeding is needed in order for professionals to implement culturally sensitive and culturally appropriate parenting-focused treatments for pediatric obesity.

COGNITIVE BEHAVIOR THERAPY

Cognitive behavior therapy (CBT) has received increasing attention as a possible effective treatment for pediatric obesity (Boisvert & Harrell, 2015; Yi et al., 2019). CBT is a theoretically based approach that highlights the connections among cognitions, feelings, and behaviors (N. R. Kang & Kwack, 2020), and it has decades of research evidence for its effectiveness in treating various psychological disorders in adults and children (APA, 2017). Specific to obesity treatment, CBT incorporates techniques involving motivational enhancement, goal setting, problem solving, and knowledge and skills that can facilitate sustainable behavior changes (N. R. Kang & Kwack, 2020). In addition, in CBT inaccurate information or maladaptive beliefs about health can be challenged and corrected; a variety of skills are modeled, taught and practiced; and strategies can be modified to help families make changes that are more consistent with health education provided and individualized for their child, family, and home environment (Bejarano et al., 2019).

Acceptance and commitment therapy (ACT) is considered a *third-wave* approach to CBT. Whereas first- and second-wave approaches focus on behaviors and cognitions, respectively, third-wave approaches focus more holistically on building skills to improve overall health and wellness (e.g., weight, hemoglobin A1c). Third-wave CBTs, including ACT, involve teaching individuals to accept aversive internal experiences rather than avoiding them, which is related to increased awareness, psychological flexibility, and behavior changes (Lawlor et al., 2020). The results of a recent systematic review were mixed regarding whether ACT led to improved weight outcomes compared with standard treatment; however, ACT did lead to significant improvements in psychological functioning for adults undergoing weight management treatment (Iturbe et al., 2022). Limited research has examined ACT for weight loss in adolescents with obesity. For example, one pilot study included six families who participated in a 16-week group-based ACT program focused on lifestyle changes (Tronieri et al., 2019). The participating adolescents experienced improvements in weight status and psychosocial outcomes, as well as hunger and physical activity. However, more research examining the efficacy and effectiveness of ACT as a treatment for obesity in children and adolescents is needed, as is an increased understanding of for whom and under what conditions it may be helpful.

CONCLUSION

Psychologists and mental health care providers trained in evidence-based behavior change strategies likely have developed skills and knowledge regarding the techniques discussed in this chapter. The key is recognizing how the treatment components reviewed can be applied to healthy lifestyle behaviors to help families and youth who are experiencing pediatric overweight and obesity as well as the physical, social, and emotional ramifications of such a chronic illness. Although research identifying critical treatment components is lacking, multicomponent treatments have decades of empirical support, and psychologists and other mental health care providers should be prepared to implement multiple strategies when treating pediatric obesity because of its chronicity and intractability. Individualizing the psychological treatments by considering the family and sociocultural context is also vital.

KEY POINTS

- Numerous strategies may be helpful for psychologists and other mental health providers to implement in pediatric obesity prevention and treatment settings.
- Many psychological strategies are included in multicomponent treatments that have been examined in research, making it hard to determine the most effective strategies and for whom and under what conditions these strategies may work.
- Individualizing psychological treatment approaches on the basis of the youth, family, and sociocultural context is critical in the prevention and treatment of pediatric obesity.

THINKING OUTSIDE THE BOX

How can obesity prevention and treatment strategies be modified to increase cultural appropriateness?

6
PREVENTION PROGRAMS

In response to increasing rates of obesity in children and adults in recent decades, and resultant calls from international organizations for obesity prevention (e.g., World Health Organization's Commission on Ending Childhood Obesity, 2017), programs for youth to prevent obesity have been developed and implemented in a variety of settings. According to the U.S. Centers for Disease Control and Prevention (2017), the spectrum of prevention includes promoting community education, educating health care providers and other professionals, changing internal policies and practices, developing coalitions and networks, mobilizing communities and neighborhoods, and influencing policy and legislation. Pediatric obesity prevention programs target numerous mechanisms thought to play a role in the development of obesity in children. They also target caregivers, family, and children at different developmental stages and in different settings.

For the purposes of this chapter, we refer to *prevention programs* generally as interventions or programs that are developed and implemented to prevent a disease or injury before it occurs, which has been identified specifically as *primary prevention* (Reisig & Wildner, 2008). A common example of primary

https://doi.org/10.1037/0000401-006
Psychological Approaches to the Treatment of Pediatric Obesity, by C. S. Lim and E. T. Burton

prevention is childhood immunizations for measles, mumps, and rubella. Specific to obesity, this could be the integration of healthier lunches and removing vending machines from public schools that sell sugary drinks and unhealthy snacks. *Secondary prevention* refers to screening for identification and treatment of asymptomatic individuals who have already developed risk factors or preclinical disease but have not yet developed the targeted condition (Reisig & Wildner, 2008). Developing a program to prevent type 2 diabetes for patients already diagnosed with pre-diabetes would be an example of this specific type of prevention program. *Tertiary prevention* has been defined as activities that manage a disease postdiagnosis to slow or stop disease progression (Reisig & Wildner, 2008). A program that targets families with a child who is overweight, with the goal of preventing the child from becoming obese, would be an example of a tertiary prevention program specific to pediatric obesity. The purpose of this chapter is to describe and review the evidence for prevention programs that target children and their caregivers with the purpose of reducing obesity prevalence (e.g., primary prevention) in a variety of settings.

HOME-BASED OBESITY PREVENTION PROGRAMS

Home-based obesity prevention programs have been developed on the basis of research indicating that the home and family environments affect obesity development in children. These programs focus on targeting the home food environment, as well as all those living in the home (e.g., other children, parents, grandparents), which potentially increases their impact. However, the findings regarding their effectiveness are mixed. A systematic review conducted by Showell and colleagues (2013) found that none of the studies included, which focused on intervening with children ages 2 to 18 years old at home, resulted in significant improvements in child weight status. However, some programs demonstrated improvements in dietary intake behaviors. Web-based programs have also been used as an obesity prevention strategy with caregivers in the home environment. Knowlden and colleagues (Knowlden & Conrad, 2018; Knowlden & Sharma, 2012; Knowlden et al., 2015) have developed a brief web-based program based on social cognitive theory for mothers of children ages 4 to 6 years that is focused on improving four healthy lifestyle behaviors (fruit and vegetable consumption, physical activity engagement, sugar-free beverage intake, and reduced screen time), and they compared outcomes with those of mothers and children in an attention-control web-based educational program. Two years after the trial, results revealed that children whose mothers had participated in the prevention program consumed significantly more fruits and vegetables compared with children whose mothers participated in the attention-control program (Knowlden & Conrad, 2018). However, no significant changes between the groups were found for the other health behaviors examined. The web-based program was designed to present information in a brief format (e.g., five modules 10–15 minutes long presented over 6 weeks), and effects were examined after 2 years in a relatively small sample size, which, taken together, could explain some of the limited findings. It could be that more intense and longer home-based prevention programs would have a greater impact on multiple health behaviors and/or weight outcomes.

SCHOOL-BASED PREVENTION PROGRAMS

Schools have been a major target for child obesity prevention. The World Health Organization's Commission on Ending Childhood Obesity (2017) identi-fied six recommendations for addressing the obesity epidemic (see Table 6.1), one of which focuses specifically on schools as an avenue to target nutrition, physical activity, and health in school-age children. The U.S. Centers for Disease Control and Prevention's (2021) Whole School, Whole Community, Whole Child model outlines the role schools play in promoting health in youth and facilitating the adaptation of health behaviors throughout childhood while recognizing that health behaviors are easier to change earlier in life. Schools

TABLE 6.1. Recommendations from the World Health Organization's Commission on Ending Childhood Obesity for Preventing and Treating Pediatric Obesity

- Use comprehensive programs that promote the intake of healthy food and reduce the intake of unhealthy foods and sugar-sweetened beverages.
- Implement comprehensive programs that promote physical activity and reduce sedentary behaviors.
- Strengthen guidance for noncommunicable disease prevention and integrate it with current guidance for preconception and prenatal care.
- Provide guidance on, and support for, a healthy diet, sleep, and physical activity in early childhood to ensure children grow appropriately and develop healthy habits.
- Implement comprehensive programs that promote healthy school environments, health and nutrition literacy, and physical activity among school-age children and adolescents.
- Provide family-based, multicomponent, lifestyle weight management services for children and young people with obesity.

Note. This table was created on the basis of information presented by the World Health Organization Commission on Ending Childhood Obesity (2017).

have been a target for prevention because of the amount of time children of varying ages spend in these settings. For example, children enrolled in day care may spend 8 to 9 hours a day in that setting, and in elementary school children may eat breakfast, lunch, and a snack during the school day. Thus, children of various ages may eat the majority of their meals in the school setting during the school week. This is a setting in which caregivers have limited control, especially if children are receiving free and reduced-price lunch or families are not able to provide food for their child to take to school. In addition, children may have classes during school days that are specific to physical education and focus on various health topics. School settings are also trusted sources of information to caregivers, especially in underresourced communities. School personnel may be viewed in some communities as important sources of child health information and can provide caregivers with education regarding healthy lifestyle behaviors targeted in obesity prevention (Robinson et al., 2019). Some child care and educational settings may be at increased risk of having students with a higher risk of developing overweight and obesity, such as publicly subsidized educational settings provided for low-income families (e.g., Head Start preschools, a federally funded program in the United States for low-income children), or those located in racially/ethnically diverse and/or underresourced communities, given that low socioeconomic status is associated with increased obesity risk and systemic racism that affects housing and educational opportunities (Fradkin et al., 2015). Taken together, this has resulted in the development of numerous forms of obesity prevention programs implemented in child-focused educational settings.

Child Care Settings

For young children, child care settings, such as day care facilities and Head Start centers, have been an avenue for the implementation of obesity prevention programs. In one systematic review, most of the programs identified targeted both nutrition and physical activity, but some focused on only one of these healthy lifestyle targets (Zhou et al., 2014). Almost half of the studies included youth from socioeconomically disadvantaged backgrounds, and some included racially/ethnically diverse children. A majority of the included studies demonstrated improvements in weight-related outcomes, and all of those that noted child weight improvements included both nutrition and physical activity components in their prevention programs. The authors of the systematic review encouraged future obesity prevention programs in child care settings to consider the built environment and ways to increase active outdoor and indoor play to increase sustainability related to engagement in physical activity. The authors also found that even when prevention interventions were culturally tailored, significant improvements in child weight outcomes or health behaviors were not found. Thus, more obesity prevention research is needed in child care settings that focuses on developing interventions to meet specific needs of young children and their families from diverse racial, cultural, and socioeconomic backgrounds. Other author recommendations were related to implementing institutional changes (e.g., changing policies, preschool staff training) and including more cost-effectiveness information to inform the sustainability potential of obesity prevention programs in the child care setting.

Some prevention programs implemented in child care settings have been developed to target specific mechanisms that lead to the development of obesity. For example, Lumeng and colleagues (2017) developed and implemented an obesity prevention program that targeted self-regulation skills in preschoolers attending Head Start, in addition to providing education about healthy lifestyle behaviors. Emotional and behavioral dysregulation are thought to increase obesity risk (Gunstad et al., 2020). More than 600 children were included in the study and, the sample was diverse in regard to race/ethnicity (e.g., 48% non-Hispanic White, 30% non-Hispanic Black, and 12% Hispanic). Although the self-regulation and lifestyle program improved teacher report of child self-regulation skills, it had no effect on obesity prevalence or on most obesity-related behaviors assessed. The authors did not examine potential differential impacts of the program based on child race/ethnicity despite them identifying child race/ethnicity as moderating the effectiveness of similar prevention programs in previous research. This is a vital future direction for obesity prevention programs implemented in early child care settings targeting racially, ethnically, and socioeconomically diverse children.

Elementary School Age

Numerous obesity prevention programs for elementary school-age children have been implemented and examined. One program trained teachers to implement a combined health and academic curriculum for second-grade students through the use of curriculum materials and teaching aides for academic and elective subjects and included the assistance of a health professional trained in motivational interviewing (Johnston et al., 2013). Students with overweight or obesity who received the teacher-led health curriculum with health professional support demonstrated significant improvements in weight status compared with students with overweight or obesity who received the health curriculum without the support of the health professional. However, the authors found no group differences in weight status in students who were not overweight or obese. This study highlights that school-based obesity prevention messages may differentially affect students on the basis of their weight status and that there is a need for prevention strategies implemented in schools to be applicable to students across the weight continuum. There is also a potential for school-based obesity prevention programs to have different effects based on race/ethnicity and culture. School-based programs vary in terms of their level of implementation (e.g., individual students, single schools, school district, state wide) and focus on a variety of health behaviors through changes in the school curriculum, environment, and policies focused on promoting healthy lifestyles (Venturelli et al., 2019). Overall, outcome findings with regard to the impact of these programs on weight status and health behaviors have been mixed, but Venturelli and colleagues emphasized the importance of examining the local impact of obesity prevention programs and their potential effects on inequalities related to socioeconomic status and subgroups of the population who are at increased risk, such as racial/ethnic minority groups.

Schools may be especially important for obesity prevention in underresourced communities, such as those that are in rural and/or poor communities. C. S. Lim and colleagues (2022) conducted a scoping review of obesity prevention programs implemented in rural school-based settings. They found that most prior programs included a combination of nutrition and physical activity components and that teachers primarily implemented the programs. The involvement of teachers and school staff is important to consider in regard to the feasibility of obesity prevention programs in school-based settings. Of the 72 articles included in the review, fewer than 20% ($n = 14$) reported improvements in weight-related outcomes. In addition, and generally in rural school-based settings, combined obesity prevention programs (e.g., those that target both eating and physical activity behaviors) that provide a high dose of prevention/intervention (e.g., length, intensity) may be the most effective at influencing weight-related outcomes. More scientifically rigorous research in this area is needed.

Middle School and High School Age

Schools have also been a place where adolescents have been targeted for obesity prevention. A review focused on adolescents (e.g., defined as those 10–19 years of age, spanning middle school and high school) found that a majority of the primary prevention programs were implemented in schools (Flodgren et al., 2020). Overall, school-based obesity prevention programs with adolescents have yielded limited evidence for improving weight status or weight-related outcomes, but some improvements in specific health behaviors, such as reducing sugary beverage consumption, which was attributed to the implementation of school policies specific to these health behaviors, have been found. Flodgren and colleagues emphasized that research examining obesity prevention programs with adolescents is limited and that the strength of the previous work in this area is weak compared with research on prevention programs geared toward younger children. Despite the amount of previous research focused on school-based obesity prevention, there is a need for continued research in this area, especially with adolescents from diverse communities.

CLINIC-BASED PREVENTION PROGRAMS

Pediatric primary care medical clinics are another potential avenue for clinic-based pediatric obesity prevention programs. This setting is important because medical providers, especially primary care pediatricians, form relationships with caregivers and children early in life and often follow children from birth until early adulthood (Fornari et al., 2021). HealthySteps, which involves enhanced developmental services and parenting support in the pediatric primary care setting, is an example of a universal practice-based prevention program (Minkovitz et al., 2007). With regard to the prevention of obesity, there has been increasing importance placed on the first 1,000 days of a child's life specific to growth and the establishment of dietary habits and later obesity risk (Baidal et al., 2016). There is also evidence that, to prevent obesity development in adulthood, prevention and treatment efforts should begin before age 6 years (Buscot et al., 2018).

Measuring child growth—specifically, weight and height relative to age and gender—at primary care well-child visits is an important first step in assessing and tracking child weight status. The U.S. Preventive Services Task Force recommends that children 6 years and older are screened for overweight and obesity (Barton & The U.S. Preventive Services Task Force, 2010). However, research suggests that approximately 25% of primary care pediatric visits with children with excess weight lacked height and weight measurements (Patel et al., 2010). Primary care pediatric offices are often under pressure related to time, space, and patient demands, and it may seem overwhelming to screen for obesity because of competing preventative and treatment-related information demands. In addition to assessing weight status and screening for obesity in youth, primary care pediatricians also provide education and anticipatory guidance about multiple areas of child development.

Medical and other health care providers typically provide caregivers with information about typical developmental milestones (e.g., talking, walking, toileting) and preventing common childhood injuries (e.g., swimming, bike helmet use, car seat use) at primary care well-child check-up visits, but feeding and eating behaviors, as well physical activity and sedentary behavior, may not be discussed if the infant or child is growing appropriately. However, education about these topics could be explicitly included in primary care visits, which would be consistent with expert recommendations for the prevention of childhood overweight and obesity (Barlow & The Expert Committee, 2007). There has also been recent recognition that anticipatory and preventative counseling about childhood obesity needs to occur at every primary care visit, starting at birth (C. L. Brown & Perrin, 2018).

The First 1000 Days intervention is an example of a systems-level program implemented in community health centers that starts in early pregnancy and follows mothers and infants until age 2 years (Blake-Lamb et al., 2018). It incorporates the following system- and individual-level components: staff and provider training with a focus on obesity prevention across early life, expanded tracking of gestational weight gain and infant weight, universal screening for health behaviors and sociocontextual factors, patient advocates to support healthy behavior change and integration of clinical and public health services, individual health coaching for mothers at increased risk for excess gestational weight gain or infant overweight, and health education and support via multimedia techniques (e.g., handouts, posters, text messages). Obesity prevention targets are related to nutrition and activity behaviors, with a specific focus on caregiver feeding practices and infant sleep, which are targeted throughout the program, starting in early pregnancy (Taveras et al., 2021). An examination of 12-month outcomes revealed that infants enrolled in First 1000 Days centers had significantly lower odds of being overweight at 6 months and 12 months of age compared with infants attending comparison community health centers. Mothers in the treatment centers also benefited, through increased engagement in postpartum medical care, suggesting that the intervention resulted in improvements for both the mother and infant.

Another example of a clinic-based prevention program was developed to focus on increasing caregiver health literacy via educational materials and medical provider training focused on health education and goal setting (Sanders et al., 2021). Caregiver–child dyads were recruited when the child was 2 months old. Weight outcomes were assessed at well-child visits and compared with those of a control group who received typical pediatric primary care. The results revealed that the prevention group had decreased weight gain at 18 months of age compared with the control group, but this improvement was not sustained when the children were age 24 months. Nevertheless, the authors concluded that these findings are clinically meaningful and provide support for health-literacy–focused prevention efforts in pediatric primary care clinics. Primary care prevention programs have also been implemented with other health care staff (e.g., nurses). In a cluster randomized controlled trial that examined a motivational interviewing approach in a pediatric primary care setting, nurses trained in motivational interviewing provided nine sessions (one group, six individual in-person sessions, and two individual phone calls) over the course of 39 months (children ranged in age from 9 months to 48 months; Döring et al., 2016). No significant differences were found in weight status between the treatment and control groups, but some treatment effects were found for certain aspects of dietary intake. Given the time limitations primary care providers face, pediatric obesity prevention programs need to be designed to be practical to implement in this setting, and more research needs to be conducted to identify ways to increase efficacy. In addition, it could be that longer periods of time to follow the weight status trajectories of youth are needed to further identify potential long-term impacts of these primary care prevention programs.

COMMUNITY-BASED PREVENTION PROGRAMS

In addition to the World Health Organization and the U.S. Centers for Disease Control and Prevention, the Institute of Medicine (2012) also recommends a comprehensive approach to childhood obesity prevention, with an emphasis on inclusion of the community. There has been an increase in the design and implementation of community-based childhood obesity prevention programs in response to calls from these international and national organizations. In a previous systematic review of community-based pediatric obesity prevention programs, 11.1% (e.g., one out of nine) of the included articles reported on research conducted exclusively in a community-based setting; all the others (e.g., 88.9%, or eight out of nine) were implemented in the community and in an additional location, such as a school, home, primary care, or child care setting (Bleich et al., 2013). Bleich and colleagues found that four of the nine studies reported improvements in child weight status, and these studies specifically used combined dietary and physical activity approaches with children (e.g., middle school age or younger) and were implemented in multiple settings.

To compare the effectiveness of childhood obesity prevention approaches in specific community-based settings, Y. Wang and colleagues (2015) conducted a systematic review and meta-analysis that included 139 articles. They concluded that there is moderate evidence for the effectiveness of community-based prevention programs, but most were conducted in school settings. With regard to the most effective combinations of components and settings, they found that interventions that included physical activity only, delivered in schools with home involvement, and interventions that combined diet and physical activity, delivered in schools with additional home and community components, were the most effective at improving weight status. *Culinary Medicine* has recently been identified as a potential avenue for the primary prevention of obesity in community-based settings. Culinary medicine has been recognized as an evidence-based field that combines food and cooking with the science of medicine (La Puma, 2016). This curriculum has been integrated at numerous academic medical centers and the program implemented in a variety of settings (e.g., food pantries, schools, community organizations) with both adults and children. For example, one pilot Culinary Medicine program designed for children whose parents were using a food pantry found that children, after participating, were able to identify new foods, more likely to want to help prepare food at home, and willing to try new foods (Marshall & Albin, 2021). Currently, there are limited published data regarding how Culinary Medicine and similar programs influence weight-related and other health outcomes in adults and youth. This would be an important avenue to explore in future obesity prevention research, as would continuing to examine the utility of these programs with families with limited resources and from diverse backgrounds as a way to address health inequities.

POLICY PREVENTION PROGRAMS

Similar to other public health issues, local, state, and national policies have been recognized as an additional way to address the obesity epidemic. For example, implementing a tax on sugary beverages is a policy approach similar to that used to reduce cigarette smoking at the population level (e.g., increased taxes on nicotine products). The World Cancer Research Fund International developed a framework called NOURISHING specific to food policies to prevent obesity through improving the availability, affordability, and acceptability of healthy foods and decreasing the availability and acceptability of unhealthy foods (Hawkes et al., 2013; see Table 6.2). This framework focuses on developing policies in the food environment, food system, and behavioral change communication domains. The World Cancer Research Fund International (2022) also developed a policy framework called MOVING, which focuses on ways to promote physical activity (see Table 6.2). The MOVING framework

TABLE 6.2. Framework for Obesity Prevention Policies From the World Cancer Research Fund International

NOURISHING food policies framework
☐ Nutrition label standards and regulations on the use of claims and implied claims on food.
☐ Offer healthy foods and set standards in public institutions and other specific settings.
☐ Use economic tools to address food affordability and purchase incentives.
☐ Restrict food advertising and other forms of commercial promotion.
☐ Improve nutritional quality of the whole food supply.
☐ Set incentives and rules to create a healthy retail and food service environment.
☐ Harness food supply chain and actions across sectors to ensure coherence with health.
☐ Inform people about food and nutrition through public awareness.
☐ Nutrition advice and counselling in health care settings.
☐ Give nutrition and education skills.

MOVING physical activity policies framework
☐ Make opportunities and initiatives that promote physical activity in schools, the community, and sport and recreation.
☐ Offer physical activity opportunities in the workplace and training in physical activity promotion across multiple professions.
☐ Visualize and enact structures and surroundings which promote physical activity.
☐ Implement transport infrastructure and opportunities that support active societies.
☐ Normalize and increase physical activity through public communication that motivates and builds behavior change skills.
☐ Give physical activity training, assessment and counselling in healthcare settings.

Note. This table was created on the basis of information presented by Hawkes et al. (2013) and the World Cancer Research Fund International (2022).

emphasizes the roles and importance of active societies, active environments, and active people across the life span. Both of these frameworks are intended to help categorize policy efforts and help policymakers individualize obesity prevention efforts specific to their local or national contexts and populations as well as to identify policy approaches that are informed by research. Psychologists and other practitioners working to develop and implement policy-based programs should keep these frameworks in mind and advocate for policies that have been informed by and developed on the basis of the available research evidence.

Research on community programs and policies focused on childhood obesity prevention in the United States has been conducted through the National Institutes of Health-funded Healthy Communities Study (National Heart, Lung, and Blood Institute, 2018), which followed 130 communities for a 10-year period to examine associations between specific characteristics of prevention policies and programs and weight and lifestyle behavior outcomes in children in kindergarten through eighth grade (Frongillo et al., 2017; Strauss et al., 2018). Frongillo and colleagues (2017) found that communities that targeted more childhood obesity prevention behaviors (e.g., physical activity and nutrition) had lower weight status outcomes, which equated to a reduction in expected childhood obesity prevalence in these communities. Thus, more intensive community- and policy-based programs resulted in lower obesity rates. There is also evidence that more community- and policy-based obesity prevention programs are associated with improvements in child dietary intake and engagement in physical activity (Pate et al., 2018; Ritchie et al., 2018; Webb et al., 2018). Additional analyses revealed that the intensity of the intervention and improvements in child weight status varied on the basis of family and community characteristics (e.g., child age, race/ethnicity, family income, and parent education; Strauss et al., 2018). Community- and policy-based approaches also differentially affect child engagement in physical activity. For example, Pate and colleagues (2018) found that more intense community- and policy-based obesity prevention programs were associated with increased physical activity, but only for non-Hispanic youth. For Hispanic youth, more intense community and policy approaches were associated with decreased engagement in physical activity. This provides additional evidence that one should consider health equity when designing community- and policy-based obesity prevention programs.

In a systematic review and meta-analyses focused on obesity prevention policies, Taghizadeh and Farhangi (2020) found that short-term school-based policies implemented with younger children (e.g., age 5–10 years) and that targeted both diet and physical activity were the most effective. More research is needed to continue to examine the impact of obesity prevention policies on children and families.

CONCLUSION

There is a body of research that has examined the efficacy and effectiveness of pediatric obesity prevention programs in a variety of settings. Much of the available research has limited findings with regard to improvements in weight-related or obesity-related outcomes, yet it is important to understand the potential impact of prevention programs on the larger population. Prevention programs not only potentially influence child weight-related outcomes, but programs conducted with and for parents or caregivers may have more significant public health impacts because of the potential for them to improve parent and caregiver health factors. For example, small to moderate impacts from prevention programs on individual weight outcomes across the population have the potential to significantly affect public health and health care expenditures, which may not be realized until a much later time (Y. Wang et al., 2015). In addition, obesity prevention programs may be influencing other outcomes not directly measured or evaluated, such as psychological functioning and quality of life, which further improve public health on a population level.

Similar to the treatment of pediatric obesity, there is a need for interdisciplinary approaches to the primary prevention of childhood obesity. Hilbert and colleagues (2008) identified both individual factors (e.g., genetics, psychology) and environmental factors (e.g., law, economics) within the context of ethics that need to be considered for the primary prevention of pediatric obesity. For pediatric obesity prevention programs to be more effective, they need to include a multidimensional approach that consists of different components (e.g., physical activity, nutrition and eating behaviors, sleep), developmental periods, levels of prevention (individual, family, community, policy), and longer durations (Fornari et al., 2021). In addition, there is a need for prevention programs that incorporate social factors that are associated with increased obesity risk in children. A number of social vulnerabilities have been identified as being associated with obesity in youth, such as growing up in a family with lower income, having caregivers who lack social support, caregiver unemployment, being from a racial/ethnic minority or immigrant background, experiencing adverse childhood events, being female, and being raised in a nontraditional family (Iguacel et al., 2021). Despite the body of evidence suggesting that these factors are important for the development of pediatric obesity, few prevention programs have been designed with reducing these specific vulnerabilities in mind. Parenting support programs and educational and occupation development programs may be potential avenues that could address some of these factors. From both a health equity and obesity prevention perspective, there is a need for social cultural factors—both risk and protective—to be integrated into pediatric obesity prevention programs. In addition, it is important for psychologists and other health care providers working with children and families to support caregivers and take a family systems approach when providing education about health behaviors— specifically, feeding/eating, physical activity, and sleep—and to provide support during pregnancy and throughout childhood to reduce childhood trauma and neglect and help caregivers learn developmentally appropriate parenting practices that can not only reduce the prevalence of pediatric obesity but also improve other public health issues (e.g., anxiety, depression, behavior problems, learning issues).

KEY POINTS

- Prevention programs that focus on multiple health behaviors and target younger children and family-system factors are likely to be the most impactful by reducing long-term obesity risk.

- More longitudinal research that examines prevention programs with economically, racially, and ethnically diverse youth is needed, as is research that includes both social-cultural risk and protective factors.

THINKING OUTSIDE THE BOX

What protective factors could be integrated into pediatric obesity prevention programs?

7 RETAIL AND IMMERSION PROGRAMS

Commercial, or retail, weight loss programs for adults are a thriving industry, estimated to be worth over $250 billion worldwide and over $72 billion in the United States alone, with these numbers expected to rise in the coming years ("The $72 Billion Weight Loss and Diet Control Market," 2019; "Global Weight Loss Products and Services Market Report 2021," 2021). More recently, retail and immersion programs have begun to target children and adolescents with overweight and obesity.

RETAIL/COMMERCIAL WEIGHT MANAGEMENT PROGRAMS

In the treatment of adults with obesity, commercial programs have been available for more than 50 years (Dietz et al., 2015). There is evidence from long-term trials that the three largest commercial programs—Jenny Craig, Nutrisystem, and WW (formerly known as Weight Watchers International, Inc.)—demonstrate benefits (Dietz et al., 2015). For example, after 12 months enrolled in these commercial programs, the average weight loss in adults

https://doi.org/10.1037/0000401-007
Psychological Approaches to the Treatment of Pediatric Obesity, by C. S. Lim and E. T. Burton

ranges from 15 to 17 lbs (7–9 kg). However, these commercial programs vary in numerous ways in regard to the structure and support provided, costs, efficacy, and scientific basis, as well as the individual's abilities to engage in long-term program adherence. Randomized controlled trials of commercial weight management programs for adults are limited, but some commercial programs have demonstrated efficacy and safety (Laudenslager et al., 2021). Researchers have started to examine the utility of commercial weight management programs for children and adolescents.

For adolescents ages 13 to 17 years, a program called JenMe was developed and implemented in Jenny Craig centers. This program was an individualized 12-week in-person program developed by dietitians at Jenny Craig (Bonham et al., 2017). The weekly individual sessions focused on dietary and behavioral education and monitoring of progress with a Jenny Craig-trained consultant. Prepackaged Jenny Craig foods were included in the individualized menus adolescents followed during the program and were supplemented with store-bought healthy foods. Bonham et al. found that, compared with a wait-list control group, adolescents who participated in the JenMe program experienced significant decreases in weight status after 12 weeks, as well as decreased intake of dietary calories and increased engagement in physical activity. This study also demonstrated significant improvements in body image and obesity-specific health-related quality of life in participating adolescents. Adolescents who took part in this study varied in socioeconomic status, but information regarding their race or ethnicity was not reported (the study was conducted in Australia). More information regarding the acceptability, feasibility, and effectiveness of the program for diverse youth would be important.

WW recently developed an application for mobile phones and other devices, called Kurbo, that was developed for use with children and teens (Cardel & Taveras, 2020). Virtual and mobile programs have the potential to be more feasible for families because of the barriers that may make attending in-person clinic visits difficult (e.g., transportation, distance and location of clinic, time off work and school). The Kurbo program consists of a mobile app for self-monitoring of eating, physical activity engagement, and weight, as well as individualized video coaching sessions by Kurbo-certified behavioral coaches (Chew et al., 2021). In an initial evaluation consisting of more than 1,000 youth 5 to 18 years of age, researchers found that youth participated in about nine weekly health coaching sessions and consistently engaged with the app to report their lifestyle behaviors (Cueto et al., 2019). In addition, they reported a relatively lower dropout rate compared with that documented for pediatric weight management in-person medical clinic visits (e.g., the overall program retention was about 80% compared with about 41% for clinic-based pediatric weight management programs; Tucker et al., 2022). Another important finding is that improvements in reported weight status were significantly associated with the number of health coaching sessions youth attended. Thus, consistent engagement in the app through its main components (self-monitoring of weight and lifestyle behaviors and engagement in health coaching) were vital for effectiveness. Sociodemographic information about participating youth and their families (e.g., race/ethnicity, family income, parent education) were not collected, so data regarding acceptability, feasibility, and effectiveness for diverse youth are not available.

Chew and colleagues (2021) have used Kurbo as an initial treatment when youth are referred to an outpatient interdisciplinary pediatric weight management program and were awaiting their initial medical appointment. During the 12-week study period, adolescents engaged in about seven individual health coaching sessions. No significant changes in weight status after 6 months were found, but there were significant improvements in body composition, dietary intake, and quality of life. This study took place in Singapore, and the sample was described as multiethnic Asian. The majority of the sample had a family income below the national median. Thus, there is some evidence for effectiveness of the Kurbo app with diverse adolescents. However, more research in other populations is warranted.

In general, commercial weight loss programs, whether in person or technology based, appear promising in the short term for the treatment of overweight and obesity in youth and may provide additional treatment avenues, especially for youth who may not have access to interdisciplinary pediatric obesity treatment centers or those from underresourced backgrounds (Cardel & Taveras, 2020); however, more research using larger samples and with longer follow-up periods are warranted to better examine outcomes, maintenance of outcomes, and potential adverse effects. Adherence and cost-effectiveness data are also needed to better understand feasibility.

IMMERSION WEIGHT MANAGEMENT PROGRAMS

Immersion weight management programs place patients with overweight or obesity in a therapeutic and educational environment for long periods of time, which removes them from obesogenic environments and restricts dietary intake, increases engagement in physical activity, and focuses on improving self-esteem (K. P. Kelly & Kirschenbaum, 2011). Immersion treatment for weight loss has been defined previously as an intervention or program involving 24-hour attendance for at least 10 days (Kirschenbaum, 2010). The television show *Biggest Loser* is an example of an intense immersive environment meant to result in weight loss for adults. In children, immersion treatments include camps, spas, inpatient or hospital settings, and boarding schools (K. P. Kelly & Kirschenbaum, 2011).

For children with overweight or obesity, the summer months are a time period prone to increased weight gain (Franckle et al., 2014). Intensive summer camp programs are one type of immersion program that have been used to combat this and to treat pediatric obesity. Summer camp immersion programs typically incorporate education about healthy eating and nutrition, regular engagement in physical activity through outdoor and sports activities, and coping skills to improve self-esteem and confidence. Several studies have examined their effectiveness at producing initial weight loss (Gately et al., 2000, 2005; Huelsing et al., 2010; Kirschenbaum et al., 2007), as well as improvements in quality of life (Patrick et al., 2011) and psychological functioning (Walker et al., 2003). However, there is limited information regarding maintenance of weight loss and dietary and physical activity changes that are initiated during a residential summer camp program. In addition, the generalizability of data from residential summer camps is limited. These programs are available only in specific parts of the country, which mean patients and their families may have to travel far distances to participate.

Many privately owned and operated residential summer camps are expensive (e.g., $3,000–$11,000 per child; https://www.campnewheights.com/dates-rates, https://www.camppoconotrails.com/moms-family-camp/) and time intensive (e.g., 2–8 weeks), which adds additional burden and costs to families. Because of these reasons, residential summer camps may be a reality for only a very small number of children with overweight or obesity, and they are not practical for dissemination and implementation in community-based settings.

Pediatric obesity-focused summer day treatment camps have also been developed and evaluated. These camps typically involve the child attending a camp during daytime hours for 6 to 8 weeks. Education about healthy nutrition and engagement in physical activities are incorporated and may include the use of an evidence-based behavioral modification system similar to that used in the Summer Treatment Program for ADHD (attention-deficit/hyperactivity disorder; Coto & Graziano, 2022; Graziano et al., 2017). Evaluations of these programs using small samples have revealed feasibility and acceptability, as well as promising results related to weight status and healthy lifestyle behaviors (Coto & Graziano, 2022; Graziano et al., 2017). However, more research with larger samples is needed, as is more information about maintenance of changes and cost-effectiveness.

Residential and hospital-based programs have also been implemented and evaluated. Deforche and colleagues (2003) described a 10-month residential program for children and adolescents with severe obesity. The program consisted of medical support, but no use of medication; moderate dietary restriction, which was defined as 1400 to 1600 kcal/day; physical activity; psychological support; and some caregiver involvement. The results revealed that after completing the program children experienced significant improvements in weight status and percent body fat outcomes. Slaney and colleagues (2012) described a school-based intensive residential program lasting 10 months that took place in a rural educational environment. In this setting there were no televisions, mobile phones, or internet access, and adolescents had to engage in manual labor (e.g., chopping wood for heating and hot water), had no access to unhealthy food, and engaged in an intensive physical activity program (e.g., running, hiking, and skiing). The results of their study, which examined data from more than 500 adolescents with overweight or obesity, revealed significant improvements in weight status for boys after participating in the program, but this was not observed for girls with overweight or obesity. Thus, residential school-based intensive programs may have differential effects based on sex/gender.

Commercial residential treatment programs focused on obesity are also available (e.g., the Elk River Treatment Program [https://elkrivertreatment. com/treatment/treating-teenage-obesity], Gem Academy [https://gema cademyaz.com/]). These programs range in length but are typically for a minimum of 6 months, with costs estimated to start at $2,000 per month. There are no published data regarding their effectiveness on weight or other outcomes. More research and examination of immersion and residential programs for pediatric weight management are needed.

CONCLUSION

Although retail and immersion programs have been in use to combat overweight and obesity in youth for numerous decades, there is limited research evidence regarding their efficacy and effectiveness in both the short and long term. For both retail and immersion programs there are concerns regarding cost-effectiveness: These programs are not typically covered by medical insurance and are cost-prohibitive for children from disadvantaged backgrounds who are at most risk for obesity and related comorbidities and have the most need for them. In addition, there are questions about the developmental appropriateness of these programs for children and adolescents; the majority of retail and immersion programs were initially developed for adults and then modified for implementation with youth. Dimensions of physical, emotional, social, and psychological development are important to consider for any program targeting children and adolescents. In addition, the level of caregiver involvement in retail and immersion programs, which vary depending on the age of youth participating, is also important to consider. Some summer camp immersion programs have begun to include maternal and family programs (e.g., https://www.camppoconotrails.com/moms-family-camp/). Caregiver involvement and implementation of healthier lifestyle behaviors has been found to improve outcomes after adolescents participated in a summer camp weight management immersion program (Hinkle et al., 2011). Sustainability of outcomes from both retail and immersion programs are also important to consider. The primary role of a psychologist working with children and caregivers considering using these programs would be to educate them regarding the available research evidence, as well as pros and cons of these approaches, so families can make informed decisions. There should also be considerations of how retail and immersion programs may serve as an adjunct or supplement to care provided in interdisciplinary pediatric weight management programs. Psychologists should also discuss and make plans for helping families sustain changes to lifestyle behaviors after discontinuation or discharge from retail and immersion programs.

KEY POINTS

- Retail and immersion weight management programs may be of interest to some children and their families. Efficacy and cost-effectiveness information is currently limited, but these programs may help supplement care for those living in underresourced communities or those from diverse backgrounds.

- Psychologists should be prepared to discuss the benefits and drawbacks of these programs with youth and their families, as well as support families before, during, and after participating in retail and immersion weight management programs.

THINKING OUTSIDE THE BOX

What are ways to increase access to retail and immersion programs for youth from financially underresourced backgrounds?

8 WEIGHT LOSS MEDICATIONS

Behavioral lifestyle modification, which includes a focus on diet, exercise, and health behavior, is the first-line treatment for obesity in children and adolescents. These interventions often entail strategies to implement and maintain changes to eating and activity patterns. In light of increased risk for medical (e.g., type 2 diabetes, hypertension, orthopedic dysfunction) and psychological (e.g., depression, anxiety, self-esteem concerns) comorbidities (Pulgarón, 2013; Skinner et al., 2015), many experts assert that there is a window of time in which the deleterious effects of obesity are more reversible, and therefore they advocate for earlier intervention efforts (Hampl et al., 2023a).

In 2010, the U.S. Preventative Services Task Force (Whitlock et al., 2010) commissioned a systematic review in which they concluded that comprehensive behavioral lifestyle modification interventions require medium- (26–75 hours) to high-intensity (>75 hours) contact with providers in order to attain modest improvements in weight status (a mean change in BMI of 1.9–3.3 kg/m² after 6–12 months). The results also indicated that weight loss can be maintained over the 12 months following treatment with no adverse effects. However, lifestyle modification alone may not be sufficient for all youth, in particular those with severe obesity (Spear et al., 2007). In fact, the task force's review found

https://doi.org/10.1037/0000401-008
Psychological Approaches to the Treatment of Pediatric Obesity, by C. S. Lim and E. T. Burton

that combining medication treatment with behavioral intervention provides benefits that are superior to behavioral lifestyle modification alone (Whitlock et al., 2010).

MEDICATIONS FOR THE TREATMENT OF PEDIATRIC OBESITY

The American Academy of Pediatrics recently recommended that pediatricians should offer weight loss medications to children ages 12 and up with obesity (Hampl et al., 2023a). Despite the urgency to address obesity and associated comorbidities early in the disease process, the use of medications to treat excess weight in children and adolescents remains controversial (C. E. Thomas et al., 2016). To date, the U.S. Food and Drug Administration (FDA) has approved fewer than 10 prescription medications to manage obesity, and at present only 4 have been approved to treat obesity in children 12 years or older: orlistat (Xenical, Alli), liraglutide (Saxenda), semaglutide (Wegovy), and a combination of phentermine and topiramate (i.e., Qsymia; see Table 8.1).

Phentermine (Lomaira, Adipex-P) is approved for use in adolescents who are at least 16 years old, and setmelanotide (IMCIVREE) is approved for children 6 years and older with obesity caused by a rare genetic disorder affecting the melanocortin-4 receptor (MC4R) pathway, which is linked to appetite control (Pomeroy et al., 2021). Sibutramine (Meridia), which was previously approved by the FDA for the treatment of obesity in children 12 years and older, is no longer available in the United States because of the risk for adverse cardiovascular effects (Scheen, 2011).

In addition to FDA-approved medications, medical clinicians may prescribe medications *off-label*, or in ways that differ from what the FDA has approved (A. S. Kelly et al., 2016). Off-label uses include prescribing medications for different medical concerns than originally indicated, using multiple medications at one time, or prescribing medications for individuals younger than the age range of approval. Prescribers considering off-label medication for the treatment of pediatric obesity are encouraged to evaluate clinical presentation, medical comorbidities, family history, and social history to inform a risk–benefit ratio (Srivastava et al., 2019). The most common off-label anti-obesity medications prescribed for children and adolescent are metformin (Glucophage, Fortamet, Glumetza) and topiramate (Topamax; see Table 8.2; Czepiel et al., 2020). Stimulant medications, such as lisdexamfetamine dimesylate (Vyvanse), are also prescribed off-label for appetite suppression and reduction in binge eating symptoms. (Although this medication is approved to treat binge eating disorder in adults, prescribing it to children and adolescents for this presentation is still considered off-label use; McElroy et al., 2015.)

TABLE 8.1. Weight-Loss Medications for Children and Adolescents

Medication name (generic: brand)	How the medication works	How the medication is administered	Common side effects	Psychological considerations
Orlistat • Xenical (prescription formulation) • Alli (over-the-counter formulation)	This intestinal lipase inhibitor blocks the body from absorbing approximately one-third of fat eaten.	Orlistat is taken orally as a capsule up to three times each day with main meals that contain fat. Because orlistat makes it harder for the body to absorb vitamins A, D, E, and K, a multivitamin is also recommended within 2 hours of taking the medication.	Side effects of orlistat include abdominal cramping, diarrhea, oily stool, increased flatulence, and fecal incontinence. Side effects may worsen when high-fat foods are consumed.	Because of the undesirable gastrointestinal side effects, orlistat has been shown to have a high rate of discontinuation in young people (Sun et al., 2014).
Liraglutide • Saxenda (higher dosage of liraglutide prescribed for weight loss) • Victoza (lower dosage of liraglutide prescribed for type 2 diabetes)	Saxenda mimics the appetite-regulating hormone glucagon-like peptide-1 (GLP-1), which can lead to weight loss through decreased calorie intake. The medication should be used with a reduced-calorie diet and increased exercise.	Saxenda is injected once daily into the stomach, thigh, or upper arm. The injection is subcutaneous; it should not be injected into a vein or muscle.	Side effects of Saxenda include nausea, diarrhea, vomiting, abdominal pain, low blood sugar, headache, fatigue, and fever. Injection sites should be rotated to reduce risk of lumps under the skin.	Additional side effects of Saxenda include depression or thoughts of suicide. This medication should not be administered to youth with a history of suicide attempts or active suicidal ideation. Saxenda should be discontinued for youth who experience suicidal thoughts or behaviors.

(continues)

Table 8.1. Weight-Loss Medications for Children and Adolescents (Continued)

Medication name (generic: brand)	How the medication works	How the medication is administered	Common side effects	Psychological considerations
Semaglutide • Wegovy (higher dosage of semaglutide prescribed for weight loss) • Ozempic (lower dosage of semaglutide prescribed for type 2 diabetes)	Wegovy mimics the appetite-regulating hormone GLP-1, which targets areas of the brain that help regulate appetite. The medication also slows emptying of the stomach, which prolongs feelings of fullness. The medication should be used with a reduced-calorie diet and increased exercise.	Wegovy is injected sub-cutaneously once weekly into the stomach, thigh, or upper arm. The injection should be administered on the same day each week.	Side effects of Wegovy include nausea, vomiting, diarrhea, abdominal pain, and belching.	Wegovy should not be administered to youth with a history of suicide attempts or active suicidal ideation. The medication should be discontinued for youth who experience suicidal thoughts or behaviors.
Phentermine and topiramate • Qsymia	Qsymia combines an appetite suppressant (phentermine) and anticonvulsant (topiramate) to target weight loss. Although the exact weight loss mechanism is not known, this medication likely works by decreasing appetite, producing early satiety, and increasing the amount of energy used by the body.	Qsymia is taken orally as a pill once daily, typically in the morning. This extended-release pill should not be chewed or crushed.	Side effects of Qsymia include insomnia, dry mouth, dizziness, tingling in hands and feet, and increased heart rate. The medication may also slow the increase in height of children and adolescents.	Qsymia can be habit forming, and sudden discontinuation of the medication can lead to seizure activity. In addition, the medication may cause mood changes and suicidal thoughts.

Phentermine	Phentermine is FDA approved for adolescents ages 16 years and older. This appetite suppressant stimulates the release of norepinephrine, dopamine, and serotonin in the brain to induce satiety and slow metabolic rate.	Phentermine is taken orally as a tablet or capsule. Lomaira is typically prescribed three times daily, 30 minutes before meals. Adipex-P is typically prescribed one time per day, between 30 minutes before and 1 hour after breakfast. Phentermine is intended for short-term use, generally up to 12 weeks.	Side effects of phentermine include increased heart rate, increased blood pressure, insomnia, constipation, and diarrhea.
• Lomaira (lower dose formulation of phentermine) • Adipex-P (higher dose formulation of phentermine)			Additional side effects of phentermine include agitation, irritability, depression, and suicidal thoughts. Although phentermine can be habit forming, research shows that abuse or psychological dependence does not tend to occur in patients treated for obesity (Hendricks et al., 2014). Likewise, withdrawal does not tend to occur in patients who suddenly discontinue phentermine.

Note. FDA = U.S. Food and Drug Administration. Except where noted, all medications are approved by the FDA for children and adolescents ages 12 years and older.

TABLE 8.2. Medications Prescribed Off-Label for Weight Management in Children and Adolescents

Medication name (generic: brand)	How the medication works	How the medication is administered	Common side effects	Psychological considerations
Metformin • Glucophage • Fortamet • Glumetza	Metformin, a first-line medication for type 2 diabetes, has demonstrated a side effect of weight loss. This medication acts by lowering the amount of glucose released by the liver while helping to restore the body's response to insulin. Weight loss may be related to greater satiety, diminished hunger, and decreased food intake due to gastrointestinal distress.	Metformin is taken orally as a tablet or liquid. It is typically prescribed to be taken one to three times per day with a meal. Extended-release tablets should not be broken, crushed, or chewed.	Side effects of metformin include abdominal discomfort, diarrhea, muscle cramps, and fatigue. Abdominal distress and decreased appetite likely lend to the weight loss effect of metformin.	Behavioral side effects of metformin are rare and can include difficulty concentrating, restless sleep, and unusual sleepiness.
Topiramate • Topamax	Topiramate is an anticonvulsant used to treat certain types of seizures and migraines by decreasing abnormal brain activity. This medication has also been shown to decrease appetite, increase feelings of fullness after eating, and make foods taste less appealing, which can lead to weight loss.	Topiramate is taken orally as a tablet, extended-release capsule, or liquid. It should be taken around the same time each day.	Side effects of topiramate include memory problems, difficulty concentrating, fatigue, and diarrhea.	Additional side effects of topiramate include confusion, agitation, dizziness, and disorientation. There is also a risk of developing suicidal thoughts and behaviors when taking topiramate.

Lisdexamfetamine dimesylate • Vyvanse	Lisdexamfetamine dimesylate is a central nervous system stimulant and first-line medication for ADHD in adults and children age 6 years and older. It is also approved to treat binge eating disorder in adults. The medication increases dopamine and reduces impulsivity and inattention that may contribute to loss-of-control eating. A common side effect is loss of appetite, which can lead to weight loss. Lisdexamfetamine dimesylate should not be prescribed for weight loss.	Lisdexamfetamine dimesylate is taken orally as a capsule or chewable tablet. This medication should be taken in the morning as it may cause difficulty falling asleep or staying asleep.	Side effects of lisdexamfetamine dimesylate include dry mouth, nausea, diarrhea, constipation, headache, increased heart rate, jittery feelings, and trouble sleeping.	Additional side effects of lisdexamfetamine dimesylate include anxiety and irritability. Rare but serious side effects include mania and psychosis. There is a high potential for substance abuse.

Note. FDA = U.S. Food and Drug Administration; ADHD = attention-deficit/hyperactivity disorder.

Czepiel and colleagues (2020) suggested that hesitancy to prescribe anti-obesity medications for children and adolescents is due, in large part, to a lack of definitive guidelines governing their use. For example, the Expert Panel on Integrated Guidelines for Cardiovascular Health and Risk Reduction in Children and Adolescents and the National Heart, Lung, and Blood Institute (2011) recommend pharmacotherapy only as a final option after a youth has not lost weight through behavioral lifestyle modification. Similarly, the Endocrine Society Clinical Practice Guideline (Styne et al., 2017, p. 731) suggests that weight loss medications be administered only in conjunction with a "lifestyle modification program of the highest intensity available." Definitive guidelines, however, require strong evidence of efficacy and safety in the pediatric population; such evidence is still sparse (Borzutzky et al., 2021). This is particularly the case for medications used off-label for treatment of pediatric obesity, because data on utilization and outcomes are limited (Czepiel et al., 2020).

HOW WEIGHT LOSS MEDICATIONS WORK

Weight loss medications traditionally have tended to work in one of two ways. First, most of them act to curb or suppress appetite, leading a person to feel less hungry or feel full faster. Phentermine, the most widely prescribed appetite suppressant in adults, is approved for adolescents age 16 years and older (Ryder et al., 2017). Other medications, such as orlistat, work in the digestive tract to make it harder for the body to absorb fat from foods eaten. These medications tend to be prescribed for a short period of time, typically no more than 12 weeks. Safety and efficacy of longer term use has not been well studied and constitutes off-label usage.

Another pathway to weight loss receiving recent research and clinical attention is to target intestinal hormones (Sherafat-Kazemzadeh et al., 2013). Glucagon-like peptide-1 (GLP-1) is a hormone that is secreted when blood sugar levels begin to rise after food consumption. GLP-1 stimulates the body to produce insulin, which helps to lower blood sugar levels (Drucker, 2022). The most recently approved medications for weight loss in children and adolescents, including Saxenda (liraglutide) and Wegovy (semaglutide), are GLP-1 receptor agonists, meaning that they mimic the action of GLP-1 (see Table 8.1). In addition, these medications seem to help curb hunger by slowing the emptying of food from the stomach into the small intestine, which results in feeling full faster and longer. It is important to note that GLP-1 receptor agonists were originally approved to help manage blood sugar levels in individuals diagnosed with type 2 diabetes. Upon noting the weight loss effect of these medications, drugmakers rebranded these GLP-1 agonists for that purpose. Type 2 diabetes medications Victoza (liraglutide) and Ozempic (semaglutide) are actually the same drug as Saxenda and Wegovy, respectively, but different dosages (see Table 4.1). Prescription of Victoza and Ozempic for weight loss is considered off-label use.

Ghrelin and leptin are two hormones that help regulate food intake in the human body (Klok et al., 2007). Ghrelin is known as the *hunger hormone*, and leptin has been called the *satiety hormone*. One of ghrelin's many functions is to stimulate appetite, increase food intake, and promote fat storage. This hormone signals the brain to become hungry and seek out food. Conversely, a major role of leptin is to regulate energy balance by inhibiting hunger. In other words, leptin sends the brain a signal to stop eating when the body does not need additional energy. Proponents of this pathway suggest that anti-obesity medications, instead of focusing on appetite, should focus on balancing leptin levels (Greenway, 2015).

One such medication is setmelanotide (IMCIVREE), which acts by activating the leptin–melanocortin pathway to promote weight loss by decreasing appetite and caloric intake and increasing energy expenditure (Clément et al., 2020). Setmelanotide is approved for children ages 6 years and older with obesity due to rare genetic conditions such as pro-opiomelanocortin (POMC) deficiency, proprotein convertase subtilisin/kexin type 1 (PCSK1) deficiency, leptin receptor deficiency, or Bardet–Biedl syndrome. This daily subcutaneous injection must be continued regularly to maintain weight loss. Common side effects include skin darkening, gastrointestinal distress, and fatigue.

Research shows that a 10% weight loss is clinically significant and improves chronic disease risk factors (Ryan & Yockey, 2017). Trials that led to FDA approval for GLP-1 receptor agonists for the treatment of obesity in children and adolescents revealed that these medications contribute to significant weight loss, up to 16% for Wegovy (Weghuber et al., 2022). As development of GLP-1 receptor agonists continues, drugmakers are also targeting another hormone, glucose-dependent insulinotropic polypeptide (GIP), which helps the body break down sugar and fat. Although such medications are currently in various stages of development, trials of tirzepatide (Mounjaro for treatment of type 2 diabetes and Zepbound for treatment of obesity) and retatrutide (which is still under FDA review) demonstrate strong weight loss outcomes of up to 24% of body weight, rivaling the results of Wegovy (Harris, 2023; Rosenstock et al., 2023).

ACCESS ISSUES

Despite promising outcomes, access to newer and more effective medications is limited (Levi et al., 2023). In the months following the approval of Wegovy, demand outpaced production, and the FDA listed semaglutide (the active ingredient in Wegovy and Ozempic) on its drug shortage list.

This global shortage meant that many patients were unable to fill prescriptions, and others who had started the medication were unable to get their prescriptions refilled. It is speculated that the shortage was exacerbated by popularity owing to increased media, celebrity, and social media influencer attention (Keating & Wild, 2023), which led to widespread off-label use (people seeking weight loss with no medical indication). The shortage has also led to a black market for semaglutide, which, in conjunction with misinformation available online, makes youth particularly vulnerable to deleterious outcomes (Burki, 2022).

Access to anti-obesity medications is also affected at the prescriber level. Prescribing clinicians are charged with aligning treatment recommendations with patient preferences, presenting health concerns, and anticipated outcomes. In addition to these considerations, prescriber training to acknowledge implicit and explicit biases against patients with obesity or from underserved socioeconomic and racial/ethnic groups is an important step in addressing inequitable prescribing of weight loss medications (Wright et al., 2023).

Another important factor affecting access is financial. The out-of-pocket cost for Wegovy is estimated to be $1,400 per month. Because of the novelty of these medications, less expensive generic options are not available. Therefore, if not covered by insurance, the long-term costs can be prohibitive. However, as popularity waxes (there were approximately 135,000 new Wegovy prescriptions per week in May 2023; Wingrave, 2023), health insurance payors are more hesitant to cover the costs. Some private health care plans limit the use of Wegovy or do not offer coverage at all, and only 16 states in the United States currently cover anti-obesity medications under Medicaid plans for patients with low incomes.

It is important to note that intensive weight management treatments, including medications and surgery, still rely on behavioral lifestyle management (Hampl et al., 2023a). In other words, access to nutritious foods and safe spaces for exercise is key. The groups most affected by obesity and its comorbidities reflect the racial/ethnic and socioeconomic disparities that limit access to these medications. Long-term solutions to these access issues are critical. Research shows that people who stopped taking Wegovy or Ozempic re-gained up to two-thirds of the weight they lost while on the medication (Wilding et al., 2022). Moreover, other health improvements (e.g., markers of type 2 diabetes and hypertension) also reverted after discontinuation. Research suggests that many of the most effective weight loss medications can be manufactured and sold for 20 times less than current prices and still yield a profit margin (Levi et al., 2023). Such changes to improve access will require tremendous advocacy efforts.

PSYCHOLOGICAL CONSIDERATIONS FOR WEIGHT LOSS MEDICATIONS

Despite the recent advances in the pharmacological treatment of pediatric obesity, medications simply will not work if they are not taken as prescribed. In fact, studies suggest that fewer than half of children and adolescents are adherent to prescribed medication regimens (Rapoff & Rapoff, 2010). Researchers have identified multiple individual-, family-, and community-level barriers to medication adherence among children and adolescents (Plevinsky, Young, et al., 2020). Among these are time management, forgetfulness, stressful life events, less family involvement in treatment responsibilities, and lack of access to medications (Carbone et al., 2013; McGrady & Hommel, 2013). Other barriers include actual or perceived interference with preferred activities, adverse taste or smell of medication, pill swallowing difficulties, and injection fears (Matsui, 2007; Taddio et al., 2022). Young people with more persistent disease duration also demonstrate poorer adherence, and adherence tends to decline over time (J. L. Lee et al., 2014).

Numerous interventions have been developed to improve adherence to medical regimens (Pai & McGrady, 2014; Plevinsky, Gutierrez-Colina, et al., 2020), although few have focused on pediatric obesity. Considering that the most efficacious treatments to date are daily (e.g., Saxenda) or weekly (e.g., Wegovy) injections, it seems that needle avoidance and phobia are particularly important adherence barriers to address.[1] Furthermore, treatment knowledge is positively associated with adherence, suggesting that when children and adolescents understand the rationale and function of their medication regimen, they are more likely to adhere (Carbone et al., 2013). Psychoeducation around why medications are prescribed and how they work to manage pediatric obesity and its comorbidities is a promising next step in improving treatment adherence.

---

[1] It is important to note that at the time of this writing, oral forms of semaglutide are under development. Rybelsus, a once-a-day oral tablet form of semaglutide, has been approved by the FDA to improve blood sugar control in adults with type 2 diabetes. This medication is not approved for weight loss. With similar efficacy and tolerability profiles (Chubb et al., 2021), oral semaglutide may be advantageous for patients who are averse to injections.

CONCLUSION

Although medication management is often considered the domain of physicians and medical practitioners, psychologists and behavioral health specialists certainly play an important role. As seen in Tables 8.1 and 8.2, many of the medications prescribed for weight loss in children and adolescents carry warnings for depression and suicidality. The need for assessment and continued monitoring of mental health concerns underscores the importance of behavioral health specialists as part of a comprehensive interdisciplinary approach to treating pediatric obesity. From administration concerns (e.g., pill swallowing, injection phobias) to adherence issues, to helping combat misinformation youth may encounter, behavioral support is key to optimal outcomes from medications.

KEY POINTS

- Prescribing clinicians are encouraged to consider weight loss medications for children and adolescents with obesity as early as 12 years of age. It is imperative that developmental considerations be made on an individual-by-individual basis.

- Clinicians and patients must be mindful of the potential for weight regain once weight loss medications are discontinued.

THINKING OUTSIDE THE BOX

What are arguments for and against starting an adolescent on a weight loss medication that they may have to take for the rest of their life?

9
WEIGHT LOSS SURGERY

The rapidly increasing incidence of severe obesity among adolescents has contributed to a greater prevalence of obesity-related complications and premature mortality. Adolescents with severe obesity are at increased risk for type 2 diabetes, hypertension, dyslipidemia, obstructive sleep apnea, orthopedic dysfunction, depression, and anxiety (Pulgarón, 2013; Skinner et al., 2015). In addition to physiological and psychological sequelae, youth with severe obesity are also more likely to experience weight-based stigma and overall impairment in quality of life (Modi et al., 2008; Pont et al., 2017).

Obesity and related comorbidities that occur during adolescence tend to persist into adulthood, underscoring the public health implications of this chronic health condition (Burton, Mackey, et al., 2020; Greenberg, 2013; Skinner et al., 2018). Although lifestyle modification (i.e., dietary and exercise changes) remains the first-line treatment for adolescent obesity, current evidence suggests that such interventions rarely lead to sufficient or sustained improvement in health outcomes (Andela et al., 2019; Kirk et al., 2022). Recent clinical practice guidelines for the treatment of pediatric obesity recommend earlier and more aggressive intervention efforts, including pharmacotherapy and surgery (Hampl et al., 2023a). Advances in weight loss medications are

https://doi.org/10.1037/0000401-009
Psychological Approaches to the Treatment of Pediatric Obesity, by C. S. Lim and E. T. Burton

discussed in Chapter 8. In the present chapter, we review weight loss surgery as an intervention for pediatric obesity.

METABOLIC AND BARIATRIC SURGERY

Metabolic and bariatric surgery, often referred to as *bariatric surgery*, is a safe and effective treatment for severe obesity that can lead to significant weight loss and improvement, resolution, or prevention of many weight-related comorbidities (Arterburn et al., 2020). Moreover, studies have shown that bariatric surgery may reduce the risk of premature mortality by up to 50% in adults (Adams et al., 2007). Researchers and clinicians assert that the safety profile for bariatric surgery has improved significantly over the past 20 years. In fact, experts report that bariatric surgery is as safe, or safer than, some of the most common surgeries performed in the United States, including appendectomy, gall bladder removal, and knee replacement (Aminian et al., 2015). The enhanced safety and efficacy are likely due to advancements in minimally invasive surgical techniques (e.g., laparoscopy, an operation performed through two to four small incisions and aided by a camera), formal training of bariatric surgeons, and rigorous accreditation requirements for bariatric surgery centers (Aminian & Nissen, 2020).

Bariatric surgery is an umbrella term that refers to a variety of surgical procedures, including:

- *Roux-en-Y gastric bypass*—a procedure in which the stomach is made smaller (about the size of a walnut) and then attached to the middle of the small intestine in order to limit absorption of calories.

- *Vertical (laparoscopic) sleeve gastrectomy*—a procedure in which approximately 85% of the stomach is removed and stapled to create a vertical banana-shaped tube that restricts the amount of food that can be consumed.

- *Duodenal switch*—a procedure that combines a sleeve gastrectomy with an intestinal bypass; approximately 60% to 70% of the stomach pouch is removed and the remaining tube is attached further down the digestive tract, bypassing approximately two-thirds of the small intestine. The duodenal switch, which limits the amount of food that can be consumed and absorbed, is a complex procedure that is typically reserved for people with very severe obesity.

- *Gastric banding*—a procedure that involves placing an adjustable silicone band around the upper part of the stomach to restrict the amount of food that can be consumed.

- *Intragastric balloon*—a procedure in which saline-filled balloons are temporarily placed in the stomach to restrict the amount of food that can be consumed.

- *Endoscopic sleeve gastroplasty*—an alternative, nonsurgical option for people who do not qualify for or want traditional bariatric surgery. This minimally invasive procedure involves insertion of a suturing device down the throat and into the stomach, where sutures are placed to shorten and reshape the stomach, reducing its size and volume by approximately 70%. This is also referred to as an *accordion procedure* because folds of the stomach are gathered and stitched together. Endoscopic sleeve gastroplasty is reversible for many people.

In addition to the restriction of food consumption and limitation of calorie absorption, bariatric surgery has been shown to reduce the body's production of ghrelin (a hormone that stimulates hunger) while increasing the body's production of glucagon-like peptide-1 (GLP-1; a hormone that reduces appetite, increases feelings of fullness, and stimulates secretion of insulin, thereby helping the body to use sugar in the blood for energy rather than being stored as fat). As such, the benefits of bariatric surgery go beyond weight loss and can help prevent or reverse type 2 diabetes (Arterburn et al., 2020). There is also burgeoning evidence of beneficial effects of bariatric surgery for cardiovascular outcomes (Chandrakumar et al., 2023).

Although each of the above-mentioned surgical procedures are endorsed by the American Society for Metabolic & Bariatric Surgery (ASMBS), laparoscopic sleeve gastrectomy and laparoscopic Roux-en-Y are the most commonly performed in adult and adolescent populations (Clapp et al., 2022). Because of its safety, feasibility, and efficacy, laparoscopic sleeve gastrectomy is thought to be the most commonly performed bariatric surgery performed worldwide, and it has become the most common bariatric procedure performed on adolescents (Armstrong et al., 2019; Calcaterra et al., 2021). Gastric banding and intragastric balloon procedures have not yet been approved by the U.S. Food and Drug Administration for individuals under age 18 years in the United States. Early trials of endoscopic sleeve gastroplasty have shown the procedure to be safe and efficacious in pediatric patients (Alqahtani et al., 2019).

ADOLESCENT BARIATRIC SURGERY

Despite short- and long-term data that demonstrate significant and durable weight loss, improvement or resolution of weight-related comorbidities, and low rates of postsurgical complications or death (Inge et al., 2016, 2019;

Mackey et al., 2018), adolescent bariatric surgery remains controversial (Childerhose & Tarini, 2015; Herdes et al., 2021). Proponents of surgical intervention for adolescents with severe obesity argue that bariatric surgery can be lifesaving and that withholding the procedure until adulthood as physiological, psychological, social, and economic consequences continue to mount is irresponsible (Herdes et al., 2021; Sarno et al., 2020). In fact, the 2018 update of the ASMBS Pediatric Metabolic and Bariatric Surgery Guidelines rescinded younger age restrictions by removing the recommendation of achieving adult height or pubertal maturity (as measured by Tanner staging [a scale of physical development that measures the transition from adolescence to adulthood] or bone age) before pursuing surgery (J. S. A. Pratt et al., 2018). In 2023, the American Academy of Pediatrics recommended that adolescents age 13 years and older with severe obesity (BMI ≥35 kg/m² or BMI ≥120% of the 95th percentile) should be referred to a bariatric surgery program. It is important to note that this recommendation does not imply that every adolescent referred should undergo bariatric surgery; instead, a referral is intended to increase access by allowing adolescents who meet the criteria to consider and be evaluated for bariatric surgery (Hampl et al., 2023a). Nevertheless, many pediatricians report a reluctance to refer adolescents for bariatric surgery (Sarno et al., 2020; Woolford et al., 2010), and insurance denials for surgical coverage are higher among adolescents than adults (Inge et al., 2014).

In 2019, the American Academy of Pediatrics released a policy statement in which pediatric practitioners, researchers, and policymakers were provided practice- and system-level recommendations that encouraged prompt referral of pediatric patients who meet criteria to comprehensive pediatric bariatric surgery programs (Armstrong et al., 2019). A critical aspect of these recommendations highlights the importance of shared decision making among adolescents, caregivers, and health care providers. In order to discuss referral for bariatric surgery in a knowledgeable, nonbiased, and sensitive manner, clinicians must be familiar with eligibility criteria for the procedure (Hampl et al., 2023a). Moreover, guidelines recommend that comprehensive adolescent bariatric programs include a behavioral specialist (i.e., a psychologist, psychiatrist, or licensed counselor trained to work with adolescents; Armstrong et al., 2019). Specific roles for the behavioral specialist are discussed in the next section.

Current eligibility criteria for adolescent bariatric surgery are more conservative than those used for adults. The ASMBS Pediatric Metabolic and Bariatric Surgery Guidelines (J. S. A. Pratt et al., 2018) note that adolescents should be considered for bariatric surgery when the following criteria are met:

- Class 2 obesity (BMI ≥35 kg/m² or BMI ≥120% of the 95th percentile) accompanied by major comorbidities (e.g., type 2 diabetes, high blood pressure, high cholesterol, moderate to severe obstructive sleep apnea, orthopedic dysfunction, impaired health-related quality of life)

- Class 3 obesity (BMI ≥40 kg/m² or BMI ≥140% of the 95th percentile) accompanied by less severe comorbidities (e.g., elevated blood pressure, elevated cholesterol levels, impaired functioning in activities of daily life)

Additional eligibility criteria for adolescent bariatric surgery, including psychological and psychosocial considerations, are outlined in Table 9.1.

ROLE OF THE BEHAVIORAL SPECIALIST

Behavioral specialists, including psychologists, psychiatrists, social workers, and licensed counselors, are integral members of comprehensive bariatric surgery programs. These clinicians contribute expertise to the assessment of adolescents' psychological readiness and suitability for bariatric surgery, facilitation of lifestyle behavior change pre- and postsurgery, and supporting patients and families in navigating the complex medical setting (Burton, Mackey, et al., 2020). In addition to a thorough physical evaluation prior to surgery, adolescents pursuing bariatric surgery must undergo a presurgical psychological evaluation to assess motivation, adherence, and ability to understand and articulate the risks and benefits of the procedure (Burton, Mackey, et al., 2020; Hampl et al., 2023a; Michaud et al., 2015). Adolescents' ability to implement medical, dietary, and exercise recommendations is critically important, because presurgical behaviors may predict ability to adhere to postsurgical regimens (Woolford et al., 2012). Furthermore, behavioral specialists document psychosocial concerns such as diminished health-related quality of life; child maltreatment and neglect; family function and dysfunction; and mental health issues, including mood and anxiety disorders, disordered eating patterns, and substance use (Pearl et al., 2018; J. S. A. Pratt et al., 2018).

Behavioral specialists continue to play an important role after adolescents have undergone bariatric surgery. Immediately after surgery, patients must follow a restrictive diet that includes periods of only clear liquids and soft foods, and they ultimately must adjust to an overall calorie-restricted diet (Xanthakos et al., 2020). Adolescents may also experience pain, fatigue, and changes in mood (Hoeltzel et al., 2022). Postsurgical regimens often include paying attention to protein intake, taking supplements as directed, staying adequately hydrated, and engaging in appropriate exercise. And although bariatric surgery limits the amount of food one is able to consume, adolescents may still experience cravings and urges to eat in response to emotion (Williams-Kerver et al., 2019). Table 9.2 lists cues that may help people differentiate hunger from cravings.

TABLE 9.1. Eligibility Considerations for Adolescent Bariatric Surgery

BMI (kg/m²)	Weight-Related comorbidities	Age	Developmental and psychosocial considerations	Psychological considerations
		Surgery indicated in most cases		
≥40 (140% of the 95th percentile)	Moderate[a] • Elevated blood pressure • Elevated cholesterol • Insulin resistance • Glucose intolerance • Mild OSA	Referral for evaluation at a bariatric program is recommended for adolescents age ≥13 years with severe obesity. Not every adolescent referred for evaluation will be eligible or appropriate for bariatric surgery.	• Previous attempts at weight loss (≥6 months) • Provide assent without coercion (i.e., articulate an understanding of risks and benefits) • Demonstrate understanding of pre- and postsurgical requirements • Demonstrate adherence to prescribed health regimen • Demonstrate consistent and stable social and/or familial support	• Disease-related distress • Mild/moderate depression • Mild/moderate anxiety It is recommended that adolescent candidates for bariatric surgery presenting with psychopathology be referred for appropriate mental health services. These may be internal or community referrals.
≥35 (120% of the 95th percentile)	Severe • Type 2 diabetes • Hypertension • Dyslipidemia • Moderate/severe OSA • Orthopedic dysfunction • Impaired HRQoL			

Surgery indicated in some cases: Consider with caution

30–34.9	Life threatening • Uncontrolled diabetes • Metabolic syndrome	10–12 years	Cases in which adolescent is unable to provide assent may be considered if risk of mortality is high *and* substantial social supports are in place *and* ability of the support structure to adhere to a health regimen is strong.	• Loss-of-control eating • Binge eating disorder (untreated) • Substance use

Surgery contraindicated

<30	<10 years old, very limited evidence	• Inability to provide assent • Concern for coercion (e.g., by caregiver) • Lack of demonstrated source of social support • Pregnancy	• Active bulimia nervosa • Active substance abuse • Severe depression (untreated) • Suicidality • Active psychosis

Note. This table was adapted from information presented in Burton, Mackey, et al. (2020). BMI = body mass index; OSA = obstructive sleep apnea; HRQoL = health-related quality of life.
[a]Conditions not required for eligibility, but commonly present.

TABLE 9.2. Hunger Versus Cravings

Hunger . . .	Cravings . . .
. . . is gradual	. . . are sudden
. . . is open to all different foods	. . . are typically for a specific food
. . . is patient	. . . are urgent
. . . is a response to physical needs	. . . are often felt in response to emotional cues
. . . goes away when satisfied	. . . do not go away when satisfied
. . . recognizes that eating is necessary	. . . often elicit guilt about eating

Although psychological functioning and health-related quality of life often improve after adolescents undergo bariatric surgery, research shows that pre-existing psychopathology can persist after surgery (Bolling et al., 2019; Zeller et al., 2020). Furthermore, adolescents may develop maladaptive behaviors after surgery, including substance use, risky sexual behaviors, binge eating behaviors, and suicidal ideation (Decker et al., 2022; White et al., 2023; Zeller et al., 2019, 2020). Ongoing behavioral support is particularly salient for adolescents who endorse mental health concerns during the presurgical evaluation, and continual postsurgical assessment of psychological functioning is important so that issues that may emerge in young adulthood and beyond can be identified and treated (Decker et al., 2022; Järvholm et al., 2016).

BARRIERS TO CARE

Several multilevel barriers impede equitable access to weight loss surgery. Despite mounting evidence that bariatric surgery is a safe and effective treatment option for adolescents with severe obesity, utilization rates are disproportionately low among certain groups. Most adolescents undergoing weight loss surgery are female, White, and have private insurance (Messiah et al., 2022; Perez et al., 2020). In fact, although Black and Hispanic youth experience disproportionately higher rates of severe obesity, these youth are less likely to undergo bariatric surgery than White adolescents, even after adjusting for insurance type (Perez et al., 2020; Vuong et al., 2022). Moreover, most surgeries are performed in urban teaching hospitals (Bouchard et al., 2022). This contributes to an overall lack of comprehensive data characterizing long-term outcomes among under-represented youth, thereby limiting both referral and self-selection for surgery.

The American Academy of Pediatrics has outlined strategies to address reluctance on the part of pediatric care providers to refer youth for bariatric surgery, with education about risks and benefits of the procedure topping the list (Armstrong et al., 2019). Although a perceived lack of insurance coverage persists as a reason why clinicians do not refer (Tork et al., 2015), recent research suggests that having public insurance is no reason to delay a referral for weight loss surgery (Bouchard et al., 2022; Gray et al., 2023). Furthermore, researchers are evaluating strategies to address barriers related to competing priorities, such as the high number of required appointments and long travel distances for patients living in rural locations (Alvarez et al., 2018, 2019).

CONCLUSION

Estimates indicate that from 2015 to 2018 the annual number of adolescent bariatric surgeries increased from approximately 1,400 to approximately 1,800 (Vuong et al., 2022). As both the rates of obesity and number of adolescents undergoing bariatric surgery trend upward, it will be important to ensure equitable access to this procedure. Pediatric health care clinicians must be educated on what constitutes appropriate referral for bariatric surgery, and surgical candidates, regardless of demographic background, must be informed that bariatric surgery is a safe and effective treatment for severe obesity. Behavioral health specialists play an especially important role in supporting optimal physiological and psychological outcomes given that implementation and maintenance of behavioral lifestyle changes remain key aspects of success.

KEY POINTS

- Clinicians are encouraged to refer children and adolescents with severe obesity for weight loss surgery as early as 13 years of age, although this does not mean that all referred will be suitable surgical candidates.

- Many individuals who have undergone bariatric surgery report a double stigma-stigma regarding excess weight and stigma regarding choosing to undergo weight loss surgery.

THINKING OUTSIDE THE BOX

Given the power differential between health care clinicians and patients, is shared decision making around complex medical issues truly possible?

PART III PSYCHOLOGICAL FACTORS IN PEDIATRIC OBESITY

In Part III of the book, we review developmental and psychological factors that are important to consider in the prevention and treatment of pediatric obesity. Each chapter begins with a description of a case study from the biopsychosocial perspective, reviews research and important implications regarding the specific developmental issue or psychological symptoms, and discusses the implementation and utility of specific evidence-based practices that could address the issue in the context of healthy lifestyle behaviors and the development and/or maintenance of pediatric obesity.

10 CHILD DEVELOPMENT AND DEVELOPMENTAL CONCERNS

CLINICAL CASE INTRODUCTION

Kyle is a 6-year-old non-Hispanic White male who presents to an outpatient interdisciplinary pediatric obesity clinic with his grandmother and grandfather for health and behavior intervention at the recommendation of his pediatrician because of weight gain and picky eating. Kyle's blood work, conducted by his pediatrician, revealed elevations in triglyceride levels. His body mass index at the initial psychological visit in the clinic was 28.7, which is above the 99th percentile for his age and sex and in the obese range. The family had discussed concerns regarding rapid weight gain with Kyle's pediatrician previously but have not been able to make changes to the variety of foods he eats, which led to the referral to the clinic. His grandparents report that Kyle's weight had been normal until about 1 year ago. Developmentally, he was born on time via an emergency c-section because his mother had high blood pressure. His grandparents report that

(continues)

https://doi.org/10.1037/0000401-010
Psychological Approaches to the Treatment of Pediatric Obesity, by C. S. Lim and E. T. Burton

CLINICAL CASE INTRODUCTION (*Continued*)

he experienced failure to thrive at about 3 months of age. He walked on time, but speech and language development were delayed and continue to be below expected levels for his age. He has a history of receiving outpatient speech therapy, as well as speech therapy at school. Kyle currently lives in an underresourced community with his maternal grandmother and grandfather, who have limited incomes due to being retired and disabled. The grandparents report that Kyle's mother lives with them on and off and has a history of incarceration. When they initially presented to the clinic, his father was incarcerated but was expected to be released soon. Kyle is currently repeating kindergarten at a public school and has an Individualized Education Plan because of his speech and reading delays. Regarding eating, his grandparents report that Kyle will eat any fruit and vegetable as long as it is a Stage 2 baby food (and only a specific brand); specifically, they report that he loves carrots and green beans and will eat fruit mixtures, especially bananas and pears. At each meal, he eats two tubs of Stage 2 baby food, usually a meat and vegetable. According to his grandparents, he initially did well when solid foods were introduced, but when he became sick with an upper respiratory infection his parents began giving him chips because he would refuse other foods. He eats chips now (specifically, Doritos or plain potato chips), and his grandparents are concerned he may be addicted to them. About a year ago, he was seen by a speech therapist specializing in feeding issues to address issues with food textures, but then he began to refuse engaging in the food trials and the family stopped attending those appointments. He does, at times, regurgitate food but mostly refuses and gets upset and tearful when nonpreferred food is presented. His grandparents also report that he sometimes spits out new foods they give him. His grandmother has tried pureeing foods at home and putting them into the brand baby food jar he prefers, but he also refused to eat that. In addition to chips, he likes cookies, which he gets at night along with milk. Kyle will also eat peanut butter from a spoon, and will eat crackers with peanut butter; he also really likes Cheez-Its and Goldfish. He typically brings his lunch to school, which includes cereal, yogurt, and milk. His grandmother used to also pack him tubs of baby food, but other kids made fun of him when they realized he was eating baby food. For dinner, they report that he typically eats one to two chicken nuggets from a specific fast-food restaurant, and French fries. The family reports that if he refuses to eat everything they present at meal times, he is given chips. His grandparents also report that his restricted eating has affected their ability to go out to eat at other restaurants. Specific to behavioral and emotional functioning,

CLINICAL CASE INTRODUCTION (Continued)

Kyle's grandparents describe him as having sensory sensitivities, specifically to textures (e.g., tags on clothes, and he refuses to wear jeans) and loud noises (e.g., thunder), and state that he also has trouble adjusting to changes in routines and demonstrates some restricted interests (e.g., collects rocks, lines up cars and trucks). They describe his mood as happy, and he is active. Socially, he was shy last school year (first year in kindergarten), but this has improved this school year as he has been playing and talking more with other children. His grandmother also expresses concerns regarding him being angry toward his mom due to her living with them on and off. They generally deny other concerns regarding his emotional and behavioral functioning.

INTRODUCTION TO CHILD DEVELOPMENT AND DEVELOPMENTAL CONCERNS

All clinical child- and adolescent-focused psychologists and mental health providers should be knowledgeable regarding aspects of typical child development along various dimensions, such as motor, speech, cognitive, behavioral, emotional, and social areas (see C. S. Lim et al., 2018, for a review of developmental progression specific to early childhood, middle childhood, and adolescence that influence health behaviors). It is also important to recognize that development is multidimensional and reciprocal in that developmental changes, milestones, and transitions in various domains also intersect and influence other domains of functioning (C. S. Lim et al., 2018). Altogether, typical development influences engagement in health behaviors, including eating and physical activity. For psychologists and mental health providers involved in pediatric obesity prevention and treatment, typical and atypical feeding and eating development and motor development are important to understand so they can use this knowledge to inform treatment approaches that are developmentally appropriate and acceptable to youth and their families. In this chapter, we review typical feeding and eating development, typical physical activity engagement, feeding and eating problems that can occur in childhood, other developmental concerns to consider, and evidence-based treatments in the context of the case study of Kyle to highlight the importance of development in the psychological treatment of pediatric obesity.

Typical Feeding/Eating Development

Feeding and eating are complex behaviors that are influenced and determined by many systems, including multiple biological systems (e.g., peripheral nervous system, mouth and throat, pulmonary/respiratory, digestive; Białek-Dratwa, Szczepanska, et al., 2022). Genetic, economic, psychological, socio-cultural, parent–child relationship, and family factors also contribute to feeding and eating behaviors in youth. Development of the complex behaviors that result in feeding and eating can be characterized as motor and cognitive skills; specific feeding skills; taste, texture, and food preferences; and appetite regulation (Infant & Toddler Forum, 2014). Table 10.1 provides a review of feeding and eating specific developmental milestones psychologists and other mental health professionals should consider when focused on obesity prevention and treatment with youth.

One aspect of typical development related to feeding and eating that is important for caregivers, as well as medical and mental health providers, to be aware of is *food neophobia*. Food neophobia has been recognized as the rejection or reluctance to try new and/or unfamiliar foods (Białek-Dratwa, Szczepanska, et al., 2022). The onset of food neophobia, which is thought to begin after 12 months of age and peak between 2 to 8 years of age, is a normal developmental stage and should resolve naturally throughout childhood (Białek-Dratwa, Szczepanska, et al., 2022; Infant & Toddler Forum, 2014). However, caregiver behaviors in the context of infant and child feeding, as well as caregiver responses to child eating behaviors, are also important to consider given that caregiver behaviors can both positively and negatively influence development in various ways (e.g., parenting behaviors limiting progression to more advanced stages or moving to a more advanced stage too quickly).

Caregiver feeding behavior has been the focus of research and theoretical models for numerous decades. Researchers have posited that breastfeeding and caregiver modeling of feeding behaviors in the toddler years play significant roles in establishing long-term child eating behaviors (Birch et al., 2007). For example, one pilot study found that caregivers who used food to soothe infant and toddler distress had children with higher weight status (Stifter et al., 2011), which may influence self-regulation of food intake in the future.

Parental influence on feeding and eating is also important to consider in the context of typical child development. Caregivers have most control of feeding in infancy and early childhood. When children start attending child care and elementary school, they begin to eat more meals away from caregivers. This trend continues in adolescence as changes in social development and dietary intake patterns occur. In general, adolescents spend more time with peers, eat away from home more often and are less likely to eat family

TABLE 10.1. Developmental Stages Related to Feeding and Eating

Age	General motor and cognitive skills related to feeding and eating	Specific feeding skills	Taste, texture, and food preferences	Appetite regulation skills
Birth	• Brings hand to mouth • Opens mouth in preparation to suck/feed • Uses facial expressions to indicate likes and dislikes	• Can move tongue in and out and up and down	• Sweet taste and energy-rich food preferences at birth • Strong taste preferences learned from taste of milk/formula feeds • Demonstrates preferences for known smells and tastes	• Partial regulation of caloric intake • Roots and turns in search of nipple • Cries when hungry • Cries and turns head away; sucks more slowly, and stops sucking, when full
4 months	• Holds objects, brings to mouth, and visually explores objects • Becomes attuned to interactions of others and can pick up on stressful feeding times	• Starts to hold food and bring food to mouth	• Taste preferences are rapidly learned and new foods are more easily accepted	• Opens mouth for food, watches food, reaches for food • Turns away or shows disgust or gags at disliked food • Begins to regulate energy intake
6 months		• Gag response declines • Can move food from side to side in mouth	• Recommended introduction of complementary foods • Can eat pureed and mashed foods	
8–9 months	• Sits without support • Picks up objects, such as food, with pincer grasp	• Shows interest in trying to feed self from a spoon and begins to drink from a closed cup	• Can tolerate lumpy solid foods, mashed food with soft lumps, or foods that can be bitten and dissolved • Begins to chew • Starts to understand that similar-looking foods may taste the same	• Demonstrates interest in feeding self and begins pointing to food they know they like

(continues)

TABLE 10.1. Developmental Stages Related to Feeding and Eating (Continued)

Age	General motor and cognitive skills related to feeding and eating	Specific feeding skills	Taste, texture, and food preferences	Appetite regulation skills
6–12 months		• Front teeth begin to erupt • Can bite into harder foods after teeth have erupted • Can keep most food in mouth		
12 months	• Communicates using words to ask for or names wanted foods • Recognizes food by sight, smell, and taste			• Says word for food they want • Throws food or says "no" to unwanted or disliked food • Can be distracted by toys or screens during mealtimes
14–15 months	• Imitates adult behaviors and will try a new food if tried by an adult first	• Able to feed themselves with a spoon	• Rejection of food begins	• Moves away from meal or table to signal satiety or dislike • Imitates adult eating
19 months		• Able to drink from an open cup		
2 years	• Imitates other children's behaviors	• Can handle most foods offered as part of family meal	• Neophobic response more prevalent	• Eats more in response to portion sizes
3–4 years	• Will modify food choices to be like other children		• The variety (or lack of variety) of foods consumed predicts the variety (or lack of variety) of foods consumed in later childhood and adulthood	• Some children will respond to prompts to overeat • When pressured, reduces amount eaten • Changes food preferences to be like peers • Shows preference for restricted or withheld foods

Note. This table created on the basis of information presented in Infant & Toddler Forum (2014).

meals, and consume more unhealthy and less healthy foods and beverages (Birch et al., 2007). However, family meals in adolescence are associated with a reduced risk of disordered eating behaviors (Skeer & Ballard, 2013) and a reduced risk of overweight and obesity in early adulthood (Berge, Wall, et al., 2015). Caregiver response to typical developmental changes in feeding behaviors and adolescent autonomy related to food and beverage selection and eating behaviors are all important to consider in the context of prevention as well as in the assessment and treatment of pediatric obesity.

Typical Physical Activity Development

Similar to feeding and eating, engagement in physical activity is a complex process that is determined by the development of numerous gross and fine motor skills. Psychologists and other health care providers working in pediatric obesity prevention and treatment settings need to be aware of typical motor milestones that may affect a youth's ability to engage in developmentally appropriate physical activities. The U.S. Centers for Disease Control and Prevention provides milestone checklists for children ages 2 months to 5 years (Zubler et al., 2022). The milestones were recently updated to identify what most children, which was defined as 75% or more, would be expected to be able to do at specific ages. These motor development milestones are summarized in Table 10.2. After the age of 5, there is continued advancement of both fine and gross motor skills. There is also research demonstrating that as children get older they engage in less physical activity (Sherar et al., 2007), and gender differences are present; girls have been found to generally engage in less physical activity compared with boys (Aubert et al., 2021).

Feeding/Eating Problems

During the course of typical development, disruptions in feeding and eating can occur. It is important for both medical and psychological providers working in pediatric obesity prevention and treatment settings to be aware of these potential feeding and eating problems so that appropriate assessment and treatment can be implemented. Some of the most common issues in pediatric obesity prevention and treatment settings are discussed and reviewed in the sections that follow.

Avoidant/Restrictive Food Intake Disorder

As discussed previously, as part of normal development children progress through stages where they may be considered picky eaters or have food neophobia. However, when the restriction or avoidance of food becomes severe

TABLE 10.2. Motor Milestones Related to Engagement in Physical Activity

Age	Motor milestones
2 months	• Holds head up when on stomach • Moves both arms and legs • Opens hands briefly
4 months	• Holds head up without support when being held • Holds a toy when placed in hand • Uses arms to swing at toys • Brings hands to mouth • Pushes up onto elbows/forearms when on stomach
6 months	• Rolls from tummy to back • Pushes up with straight arms when on stomach • Leans on hands to support self when sitting
9 months	• Gets to sitting position independently • Moves things from one hand to the other hand • Uses fingers to rake food toward self • Sits without support
12 months	• Pulls up to stand • Walks, holding onto furniture • Drinks from cup without a lid • Picks up things (e.g., small bits of food) between thumb and pointer finger
15 months	• Takes a few steps on own • Uses fingers to feed self some food
18 months	• Walks without holding onto anyone or anything • Scribbles • Drinks from cup without a lid and may spill sometimes • Feeds self with fingers • Tries to use a spoon • Climbs on and off couch or chair without help
2 years	• Kicks a ball • Runs • Walks (not climbs) up a few stairs with or without help • Eats with a spoon
30 months	• Uses hands to twist things (e.g., doorknobs or unscrewing lids) • Takes some clothes off by self (e.g., loosens pants or opens jacket) • Jumps off ground with both feet • Turns book pages, one at a time, when being read to
4 years	• Catches a large ball most of the time • Serves themself food or pours water, with adult supervision • Unbuttons some buttons • Holds crayons and pencil between fingers and thumb (not a fist)
5 years	• Buttons some buttons • Hops on one foot

Note. This table was created on the basis of information presented by the U.S. Centers for Disease Control and Prevention (2022c) in Zubler et al. (2022).

enough to result in failure to meet nutritional requirements for appropriate growth and development, a diagnosis of avoidant/restrictive food intake disorder (ARFID) should be considered. According to the *Diagnostic and Statistical Manual of Mental Disorders* (5th ed., text revision; American Psychiatric Association, 2022), ARFID is characterized by a persistent failure to meet appropriate nutritional and/or energy needs associated with one or more of the following: significant weight loss or failure to achieve expected weight gain or faltering growth in children, significant nutritional deficiency, dependence on enteral (tube) feeding or oral nutritional supplements, and marked disturbance in psychosocial functioning. Thus, ARFID can be diagnosed in the context of pediatric obesity when weight gain, as opposed to weight loss, has occurred and at least one of the other symptoms is present. Additional criteria include that the eating or feeding disturbance cannot be explained by a lack of available food or a cultural practice; cannot occur in the context of other eating disorders, such as anorexia nervosa or bulimia nervosa, or be characterized by an overevaluation of shape or weight; and cannot be attributed to another medical condition or mental disorder or the severity of the eating disturbance exceeds what is routinely associated with the other medical or mental condition. Additional symptomatology includes sensory sensitivity (specific food smells, textures, colors, etc.), fear of aversive events like choking or vomiting, and/or a lack of interest in food or eating (Harshman et al., 2019). The limited research on dietary consumption in youth with ARFID has revealed that, compared with healthy youth, they consume significantly more processed foods, carbohydrates, and added sugars and significantly lower protein, vegetables, and some vitamins.

The consumption pattern of these foods is consistent with increased risk of weight gain and obesity, as well as nutritional deficits. Thus, in contrast to other feeding-related disorders, ARFID can occur across the weight spectrum (Kerem et al., 2022) and can occur in pediatric patients presenting for pediatric obesity-related medical and psychological treatment.

Pica

An additional eating issue that should be evaluated and considered in the context of pediatric obesity is *pica*. The diagnostic criteria for pica include persistent eating of a nonnutritive, nonfood substance (e.g., ice, dirt, paper) for at least 1 month; eating the substance is inappropriate to the developmental level of the individual; the eating behavior is not part of a culturally supported or socially normative practice; and, if comorbid with another mental disorder or medical condition, is severe enough to warrant independent clinical attention (American Psychiatric Association, 2022). This eating behavior may be the result of compulsive craving for inedible material or be related to medical and biological issues (Leung & Hon, 2019). For example, there are decades of evidence that, in some cases, pica is the result of an iron deficiency, such as that seen in pregnant women (Esani, 2016). Research indicates that pica is most developmentally typical in children 18 months to 6 years of age (Leung & Hon, 2019). The literature examining associations and potential mechanisms to explain comorbidity between pica and obesity is limited. However, for people who report difficulties controlling their eating or insatiable hunger, ruling out pica or engagement in pica-like behaviors would be important. For example, children with rare genetic forms of obesity (e.g., Prader–Willi syndrome) may consume frozen foods, flour, starch, uncooked rice, or other food-related substances that are not typically consumed in the specific form they are ingesting. Assessing whether an individual with eating-related impulse control problems may also consume non-nutritive substances or objects would also be important. In addition, pica is more common worldwide in areas with high rates of poverty and where regular access to food may be limited; thus, it has been proposed that the ingestion of nonnutritive substances may act as a food replacement because of availability and to appease hunger. There is also the possibility that some individuals receiving treatment for eating disorders or obesity may ingest nonnutritive substances in efforts to lose or control their weight (Delaney et al., 2015). Thus, further understanding the circumstances and function of the eating behavior is important. In a case control study of more than 7,500 pediatric and adult patients, obesity was identified as a significant predictor of pica (Esani, 2016). However, more research is needed to better understand the prevalence of pica in children with overweight and obesity, as well as mechanisms that may affect these associations. Psychologists and others working in pediatric obesity prevention and treatment settings should be prepared to assess for these problematic eating behaviors.

Other Developmental Issues

In addition to ARFID and pica, there are other developmental issues that psychologists and other mental health care providers should consider when working with youth and families to prevent and treat pediatric obesity.

Developmental Delays

Developmental and cognitive delays have been recognized by The Obesity Society (2015) as a potential contributor to the developmental of obesity because of their potential impacts on both eating and physical activity behaviors. In addition, feeding problems in early childhood may be associated with developmental delays (Putnick et al., 2022). Observational studies of young children have suggested that developmental delays are associated with higher rates of obesity (Levy et al., 2019). Rates of overweight and obesity in children treated in developmental disability clinics have been estimated to be about 40% (De et al., 2008). Only a limited amount of research has examined the prevalence of developmental delays in pediatric obesity clinical settings, but an initial examination suggested that rates of developmental disabilities are higher than national prevalence data (9.50% at a pediatric obesity clinic vs. 6.99% national data; Shepherd et al., 2018). In terms of mechanisms that may explain associations between developmental delays and obesity, there is some evidence that socioeconomic risk factors related to the development of obesity in children with developmental delays differ from those for typically developing peers; specifically, for typically developing children, more economic hardship, living in more deprived neighborhoods, and female gender were significant risk factors associated with obesity at age 5 years, but these factors were not found to be significant risk factors in children with developmental delays (Emerson, 2009). More research is needed to better understand risk factors specific for the development of obesity in children with developmental delays. Genetic and biological mechanisms may be important to consider. Many of the genetic syndromes associated with obesity (e.g., Prader–Willi, Bardet–Biedl) are also characterized by developmental delays that are evident early in life. In addition, ARFID and pica are more common in children with developmental delays (American Psychiatric Association, 2022; Leung & Hon, 2019). Caregivers whose children were receiving care in a pediatric weight management clinic and had a developmental delay reported significantly more general feeding-related concerns, and they more often endorsed the idea that vegetables and healthy foods do not taste good to their child, compared with caregivers whose children did not have developmental delays and were receiving obesity treatment (Shepherd et al., 2018).

In addition to understanding how developmental delays may influence eating behaviors, it is important to recognize delays in fine and gross motor skills. The presence of delays in these areas may limit a youth's ability to engage in physical activities, which could then result in the development of overweight and obesity in childhood. For example, caregivers whose children had both obesity and developmental delays reported that their child engaged in significantly less physical activity and experienced significantly more physical activity-related barriers (specifically related to weather, safety, disability/injury, and tiredness) compared with children with obesity who did not have developmental delays (Shepherd et al., 2018). Therefore, understanding both physical limitations and child and family perceptions regarding the ways developmental disabilities affect engagement in physical activity are important to consider and discuss when developing specific healthy lifestyle goals and plans related to obesity prevention and treatment efforts. Identification of potential functional impairments related to motor, speech, cognitive, behavioral, emotional, and social development are important, especially as they relate to feeding/eating and engagement in physical activity.

The manner in which, and in what forms, information is communicated to youth with developmental delays and their families in obesity prevention and treatment settings are important to consider. Psychologists and other providers should be prepared to informally—and, in some cases, formally—assess cognitive development and then use that information to developmentally tailor educational information presented to youth about health and healthy lifestyle behaviors, as well as health behavior interventions that are implemented.

Autism Spectrum Disorder

Autism spectrum disorder (ASD) comprises a group of neurodevelopmental diseases characterized by impairments in social behavior, communication difficulties, and engagement in stereotypical behaviors (American Psychiatric Association, 2022). There is a body of literature suggesting that children with ASD are at increased risk of overweight and obesity compared with their neurotypical peers (Matheson & Douglas, 2017; Sammels et al., 2022). National surveys estimate that about 19% of youth with ASD are overweight and about 23% are obese (Healy et al., 2019). In addition, the severity of ASD-related symptoms appear to increase the risk of feeding issues (Zickgraf & Mayes, 2019) and overweight/obesity (Healy et al., 2019; Levy et al., 2019).

Numerous explanations regarding associations between ASD and overweight have been hypothesized (Matheson & Douglas, 2017). Hypotheses include:

- medications, specifically, prescription medications used to manage the behavioral symptoms of ASD, which often have side effects related to weight gain, increased appetite, and metabolic changes.

- genetic predispositions—common genes have been identified that are associated with both ASD and obesity.

- physical limitations, such as limited mobility due to poor muscle tone and posture instability that lead to engagement in more sedentary behavior.

- food selectivity and sensory integration difficulties, such as food preferences based on texture, taste, color, and shape and increased experience of food neophobia.

In fact, children with ASD are at increased risk for ARFID, and sensory sensitivities have often been attributed to this comorbidity most often in the literature

(Bourne et al., 2022). One study found that limited food preferences was the most common atypical eating behavior in children with ASD (Zickgraf & Mayes, 2019). Although more research is needed to better explore these hypotheses, psychologists working in pediatric obesity prevention and treatment settings should be aware of the unique issues facing children with ASD that may influence weight management efforts. Prevention and intervention efforts should be individually tailored to youth with developmental delays and ASD to increase applicability and effectiveness.

Evidence-Based Treatments to Consider

Numerous psychological treatments can be considered when working with patients with comorbid pediatric obesity and developmental delays and/or feeding and eating concerns and their families (see Table 10.3). Understanding general behavioral principles is important for those working in pediatric obesity prevention and treatment settings where children may present with comorbid developmental delays. Behavior therapy, which focuses on antecedents, behaviors, and consequences of specific child behavior, would be an important treatment to consider. This approach can not only help identify the function of overeating or picky eating behaviors but also pinpoint both positive and negative reinforcements of feeding and eating behaviors and then modify the environment to change the target behavior. The behavioral principle underlying *graded exposure* or an *exposure hierarchy*, which are commonly used in the treatment of anxiety and panic disorders, would also be important to consider as a technique to gradually increase consumption of healthy foods, as well as in the context of gradual engagement in physical activity. For example, an individually tailored hierarchy of healthy foods organized by "most likely to eat" to "least likely to

TABLE 10.3. Empirically Based Treatments to Consider for Feeding/Eating and/or Developmental Delays

Concern	Treatments
Picky eating or food neophobia	• Behavioral therapy • Graded exposure
Overeating	• Behavioral therapy • Graded exposure
Avoidant/restrictive food intake disorder	• Applied behavioral analysis • Food chaining
Pica	• Behavioral therapy
Autism spectrum disorders	• Applied behavioral analysis
Limited physical activity	• Graded exposure

eat" could be created in collaboration with the child and caregiver, and then the child would gradually progress along the hierarchy. This approach can also be effective at modifying eating and physical activity behavior when paired with non-food rewards or with the development of a reward system (e.g., a sticker chart).

Applied behavior analysis, whereby principles and procedures of behavior management are used to increase adaptive behavior and reduce harmful or maladaptive behavior, has been used in the treatment of problematic behaviors in children with ASD and has been applied to feeding and eating issues, such as ARFID (W. W. Fisher et al., 2021). Specific to ARFID, *food chaining*— an individually tailored treatment that aims to broaden the foods eaten by the child by focusing on similar characteristics of what is already eaten . . . and foods the treatment team, caregiver, or patient want to incorporate into the child's diet—has also been implemented (Białek-Dratwa, Szymańska, et al., 2022). For young children, or those with developmental delays, food chaining may first involve increasing familiarity with new foods through play in order to reduce anxiety; this allows the child to have positive experiences in the context of new foods being presented individually and gradually. In this approach, interdisciplinary treatment is important, especially a dietitian to assist with monitoring weight status and analyze foods that should be introduced in the food chain. In fact, interdisciplinary treatment is essential if a child has comorbid feeding and eating concerns or developmental delays with pediatric obesity. Dietitians, speech therapists, physical therapists, and occupational therapists are often vital partners in delivering and implementing treatments for children with developmental delays and/or feeding and eating concerns.

OUTCOME OF THE CLINICAL CASE

After Kyle's initial psychological evaluation, the psychology team collaborated closely with both the medical and nutrition practitioners in the interdisciplinary pediatric weight management clinic to address his excess weight and picky eating behaviors. Initial discussions with the medical providers and the family involved conceptualizing the eating issues and exploring referral options. In regard to conceptualization, given Kyle's speech delays, history of living with multiple caregivers, and inconsistent involvement of his biological parents, his picky eating and food refusal were a way he was

OUTCOME OF THE CLINICAL CASE (*Continued*)

able to communicate with his caregivers and likely one of the only aspects of his life he may have felt like he had control over. Food refusal behaviors were also a way for him to get attention from his caregivers. Treatment options that incorporated trauma-informed care were identified as being important but were also noted to be limited in the community. Given Kyle's restrictive food intake and resulting medical and nutrition-related issues, he and his family were referred to an outpatient speech therapist with specialty training and expertise in the evaluation and treatment of children with ARFID. Given the long waiting list and time it can take to be evaluated by the speech therapy team, the psychology team introduced Kyle's grandparents to aspects of behavioral family treatment to gradually target his eating behaviors; specifically, a reward system for trying new foods was developed, and his grandparents were taught *differential attention* (e.g., ignoring whining behaviors and requests Kyle made for different foods). For the reward system, the psychology team collaborated with Kyle and his grandparents to identify small daily and larger weekly rewards he could earn for trying an agreed-upon food (e.g., initially applesauce). Getting Kyle's input and giving him some control of the foods targeted was aligned with a trauma-informed approach. Specific eating behaviors targeted initially included licking the new food, putting a small bite into his mouth, chewing a small bite, and swallowing a small bite. The family was also encouraged to pair daily rewards with specific and frequent praise in order to decrease the distress Kyle and his grandparents felt during meal and snack times. The team also discussed the importance of presenting new food when Kyle was hungry and pairing new foods with preferred foods to increase the chance of success with the reward system. The skill of differential attention was discussed with his grandparents multiple times, and they shared in follow-up visits that it was difficult for them to implement because they felt sorry for Kyle and guilty for all the turmoil he had faced during his earlier childhood. They reported having a hard time not giving in to his demands and food-related requests because of what he was continuing to experience regarding his relationship with his mother and her struggles with mental health and substance abuse. The psychology team, as well as the medical and nutrition providers, reinforced to the grandparents that they were doing what they could to help Kyle with his medical and eating difficulties and ensuring he was receiving the treatment he needed. After some initial success with the reward system, Kyle was evaluated by speech therapy professionals and was diagnosed with ARFID. They recommended feeding therapy, which Kyle and his

(continues)

OUTCOME OF THE CLINICAL CASE *(Continued)*

family attended for a few sessions. Kyle's treatment course involved in-session trials of different foods and a similar reward system, implemented at home, for food trials conducted by his grandparents. Kyle's limited food intake expanded during the course of his involvement in speech therapy treatment. His family was lost to follow-up in the interdisciplinary pediatric obesity clinic (e.g., multiple canceled appointments and no-shows), but the speech therapist documented gradual improvements in his weight status during the course of his feeding treatment.

CONCLUSION

Taking into account child development in multiple domains of functioning related to the prevention and treatment of pediatric obesity is important. Specific domains, such as feeding and eating and physical activity, encompass complex behaviors that involve multiple biological and physical systems but are also influenced by cognitive, behavioral, social, and emotional functioning as well as the specific family and cultural environment. To improve the chances of success, prevention and treatment efforts to target weight management in youth should be tailored to each child's developmental level. Other issues and experiences that interact and intersect with development, such as social determinants of health and adverse childhood experiences like the ones Kyle experienced, are also important to consider and integrate into developmentally appropriate approaches. There are evidence-based treatments that may be helpful for psychologists and other mental health care providers to address developmental concerns in collaboration with interdisciplinary specialty providers to prevent and treat pediatric obesity.

KEY POINTS

- It is important for psychologists and other mental health providers to understand typical and atypical development, as well as social and family factors, that may influence the development of feeding, eating, and physical activity behaviors.
- Pediatric obesity prevention and treatment strategies should be developmentally appropriate. Many empirically supported treatments can be modified and implemented to address co-occurring developmental delays and pediatric obesity.

THINKING OUTSIDE THE BOX

What are some ways culture influences the development of feeding, eating, and physical activity behaviors?

11

INTERNALIZING SYMPTOMS AND DISORDERS

CLINICAL CASE INTRODUCTION

Charity is a 16-year-old Hispanic female who presented to an outpatient interdisciplinary pediatric weight management clinic with concerns about how her weight is affecting her overall health. Her body mass index (BMI) at this appointment was 37.10, which is above the 95th percentile for her age and sex and falls into the Class 2 obesity range. Charity was referred to the clinic by her endocrinologist, who diagnosed her with polycystic ovarian syndrome (PCOS) and is treating her for secondary amenorrhea (irregular menstrual periods). The specific reason for referral was to support Charity in implementing and maintaining healthy lifestyle behaviors.

Charity attended this intake session with her biological father and reported that she seeks help in improving her health. Her parents are separated; Charity lives with her father during the school week and with her mother on weekends and holidays. Developmentally, she was born at

(continues)

https://doi.org/10.1037/0000401-011
Psychological Approaches to the Treatment of Pediatric Obesity, by C. S. Lim and E. T. Burton

CLINICAL CASE INTRODUCTION (*Continued*)

39 weeks and reached milestones on time. Socially, she reports having plenty of friends, although she said that her peers often tease her when hair grows on her chin. Academically, Charity is an 11th-grade honors student and expresses worries about applying to college next year. Charity's father reports that he started to notice weight gain during the lockdown period of the COVID-19 pandemic. Charity agrees, stating that she was worried about the safety of her family during this time and that cooking recipes she saw on TikTok helped her slow down her thoughts and feel more in control. She also reports feeling sad about not having been able to see or spend time with her friends during the lockdown period and said that during that time, when she was not using her phone, she was napping. Three weeks ago, Charity had an intake with a child and adolescent psychiatrist who diagnosed her with generalized anxiety disorder and major depressive disorder and prescribed fluoxetine (Prozac). She reports that she has taken most doses as prescribed but complains that she does not think the medication is working.

Charity reports having made multiple attempts at engaging in healthier behaviors, including smaller portion sizes, limiting snacks, and going to the gym. She expresses that limited motivation and low energy have hindered her long-term success; she also shares that she has an active gym membership but cannot remember the last time she went. She also reports that she often stops at a convenience store for snacks on the way to or from school; she states that she consumes these snacks in her car so her parents will not know that she is eating foods that she is not allowed to have at home. Using a motivational interviewing tool, the *readiness ruler* (see Figure 11.1), Charity rates her desire to lose weight as 9 on a scale of 1 to 10. Her father, on the other hand, states that he is much more concerned about Charity's health and happiness than about how much she weighs. He reports a family history of type 2 diabetes and hypertension and says that he wants to help his daughter avoid these health conditions.

INTERNALIZING BEHAVIORS

Internalizing behaviors are those that are directed inward; they are often considered to be indicative of one's emotional state. Children and adolescents who exhibit internalizing behaviors can experience a variety of negative outcomes, although symptoms often go unnoticed or untreated, even in severe cases (Achenbach et al., 2016; L. A. Pratt et al., 2017). Internalizing

FIGURE 11.1. Readiness Rulers

Prompt: People typically have many things they would like to change in their lives. Your motivation to change behaviors can vary based on other things that are happening. Think about a specific behavior you would like to change and answer the following questions:

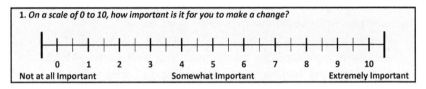

1. *On a scale of 0 to 10, how important is it for you to make a change?*

| 0 | 1 | 2 | 3 | 4 | 5 | 6 | 7 | 8 | 9 | 10 |

Not at all Important   Somewhat Important   Extremely Important

- Why are you a _____ [insert # reported] and not a zero?
- What would it take for you to get from _____ [insert # reported] to _____ [the next higher number]?

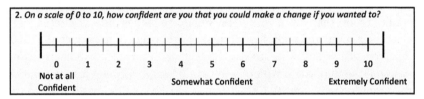

2. *On a scale of 0 to 10, how confident are you that you could make a change if you wanted to?*

| 0 | 1 | 2 | 3 | 4 | 5 | 6 | 7 | 8 | 9 | 10 |

Not at all Confident   Somewhat Confident   Extremely Confident

- Why are you a _____ [insert # reported] and not a zero?
- What would it take for you to get from _____ [insert # reported] to _____ [the next higher number]?

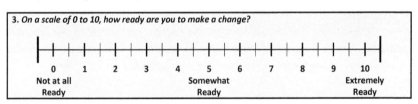

3. *On a scale of 0 to 10, how ready are you to make a change?*

| 0 | 1 | 2 | 3 | 4 | 5 | 6 | 7 | 8 | 9 | 10 |

Not at all Ready   Somewhat Ready   Extremely Ready

- Why are you a _____ [insert # reported] and not a zero?
- What would it take for you to get from _____ [insert # reported] to _____ [the next higher number]?

behaviors in childhood are associated with greater risk of poor academic achievement, poor social functioning, and future psychological problems (Graber, 2004).

The association between pediatric obesity and internalizing behaviors is complex, and research findings vary on the basis of many factors, including age, sex, familial context, and severity of obesity (E. Goodman & Whitaker, 2002; Rankin et al., 2016). For example, socioeconomic status is a predictor of obesity status, as are depression and anxiety, making it difficult to untangle the contributors to psychological functioning (Marcus et al., 2022). Another timely example from the extant research suggests that increased child and adolescent engagement with smartphones and social media may elevate risks for body dissatisfaction, low self-esteem, psychological distress, and disordered eating (Bozzola et al., 2022; Calpbinici & Tas Arslan, 2019; Girela-Serrano et al., 2022). Again, the linkages between sedentary time and excess weight (J. A. Mitchell et al., 2017) confound the relationship between pediatric obesity and internalizing behaviors.

Whether obesity is a cause or consequence of psychological distress is unclear; there is evidence that the relationship is bidirectional (Mühlig et al., 2016). Nevertheless, there is substantial empirical association between excess weight and issues such as body dissatisfaction, low self-esteem, and impaired quality of life (Rankin et al., 2016). Children and adolescents with obesity are also more susceptible to teasing and bullying, which may predispose them to anxiety, depression, and behavior problems (Gibson et al., 2017). Some studies report that youth with obesity endorse higher rates of internalizing symptoms compared with their normal-weight peers (Lindberg et al., 2020; Pulgarón, 2013), and other studies suggest that the prevalence of internalizing symptoms among youth with obesity is only marginally greater than among the general population (B. I. Goldstein et al., 2008). Findings regarding the relationship between severity of pediatric obesity and internalizing behaviors are more clear: Research reveals that, as weight increases in children and adolescents, so do their reports of psychosocial distress (Gibson et al., 2008; Phillips et al., 2012).

In the following sections, we review the current research on associations of pediatric obesity with specific internalizing disorders. Evidence-based clinical intervention strategies for these intersecting conditions are discussed.

Depression

The relationship between pediatric obesity and depression is reciprocal such that obesity predicts depressive symptoms and depression increases the risk of obesity (Kalarchian & Marcus, 2012). Several mechanisms have been hypothesized to explain the commonalities in depression and obesity. Among them are increased inflammation (higher levels of pro-inflammatory cytokines), neuroendocrine factors (lower levels of circulating brain-derived neurotrophic factor [BDNF]), and dysregulated stress system (down-regulation of the hypothalamic-pituitary-adrenocortical [HPA] axis; Bornstein et al., 2006; Luppino et al., 2010; Singh et al., 2019; Su et al., 2011).

Children with obesity often experience weight bias and stigma in the forms of teasing, bullying, ostracism, and invalidation (Pont et al., 2017). Such experiences can lead to depressed mood, social withdrawal, and decreased interest in enjoyable activities. Moreover, depression and obesity share a number of symptoms, including the following:

- Changes in appetite
  - Changes in appetite, whether an increased or a decreased desire to eat, is a core symptom of depression (American Psychiatric Association, 2022).
  - Increased appetite may lead to increased food intake and weight gain over time. In addition, food cravings may develop during depressive episodes; some patients report specific cravings for carbohydrates (that likely are due to carbohydrate consumption increasing serotonin levels; Reeves et al., 2008).
  - Youth with obesity are less sensitive to leptin, the satiety hormone that signals the brain to stop eating when the body does not need additional energy from food. In other words, leptin insensitivity can lead to increased appetite (Greenway, 2015).

- Dysregulated sleep patterns
  - Changes to sleep patterns, whether sleeping more or less than typical, is a core symptom of depression (Achenbach et al., 2016).
  - Obstructive sleep apnea, a common comorbidity of obesity, can contribute to decreased sleep at night and increased sleepiness during the day. Sedentary time and excessive electronic screen time, also predictors of childhood obesity, can likewise contribute to sleep dysregulation (Buchanan et al., 2016; J. A. Mitchell et al., 2017).

- Amotivation and inactivity
  - Decreased interest, lack of motivation, and diminished energy are core symptoms of depression (American Psychiatric Association, 2022).
  - Lack of motivation can affect readiness to engage in healthy lifestyle behaviors.
  - Sedentary time and excessive electronic screen time can decrease engagement in physical activity and overall energy expenditure (Buchanan et al., 2016; Reeves et al., 2008).

- Negative self-image
  - Guilt, shame, and a negative self-image are core features of depression (American Psychiatric Association, 2022).
  - Youth with obesity tend to report lower self-esteem and higher body dissatisfaction compared with their normal-weight peers (Franklin et al., 2006; A. Taylor et al., 2012). A negative self-image may be exacerbated by experiences of weight bias and stigma.

It is important to note that depression has been shown to play a challenging role during pediatric obesity treatment. Patients with depression tend to lose less weight and are more likely to discontinue treatment early (Jelalian et al., 2007; Taner et al., 2009). Similarly, irritability, a common manifestation of depression among children and adolescents (American Psychiatric Association, 2022), can come across as disinterest, resistance, defiance, or a lack of engagement in treatment.

Anxiety

Anxiety is one of the most common psychological disorders of childhood and adolescence (Merikangas et al., 2009). *Anxiety* can describe fear and worry and can manifest in many ways, including difficulty sleeping; school avoidance; and somatic complaints such as headaches, stomachaches, and fatigue. As with other internalizing disorders, the relationship between anxiety and pediatric obesity is bidirectional: Anxiety and strategies to cope can foster weight gain, and excess weight can contribute to social problems such as teasing, bullying, and stigma, which then can lead to increased anxiety (Grammer et al., 2018).

The link between anxiety and obesity is complex and indirect. Researchers have identified several mechanisms that may explain the association, including loss-of-control eating (see Chapter 13). C. S. Lim and colleagues (2015) found that youth with obesity who endorsed clinically significant levels of anxiety had poorer social skills than their peers without anxiety. Taken together, these findings suggest that children and adolescents who do not possess adaptive strategies to manage negative feedback from their social environment may resort to other, perhaps maladaptive coping strategies.

Anxiety diagnoses include generalized anxiety, phobias, obsessive-compulsive disorders, and social anxiety. *Social anxiety*, defined as a fear of negative evaluation and judgment by others, can affect how children and adolescents interact with their environment (American Psychiatric Association, 2022). The misdirected belief that criticism and shaming will motivate children to lose weight leads to children and adolescents with obesity often being subjected to stigmatizing language and actions (Palad et al., 2019). Youth with obesity who internalize insecurities about the physical appearance of their bodies on the basis of social norms may be hesitant to eat in front of others, apprehensive about engaging in exercise, or reluctant to interact with health care professionals. Moreover, research suggests that negative emotional states such as anxiety can also lead to emotional eating and overeating (Efe et al., 2020). A recent study of treatment-seeking youth in a pediatric weight management clinic revealed that fear of negative evaluation was associated with greater preoccupation with food, a possible precursor to disordered eating behaviors (L. M. Anderson et al., 2020).

Adult studies that have examined the links among obesity, elevated inflammation, and insulin resistance have found that social anxiety may play a key role (Jaremka & Pacanowski, 2019). Relatedly, trauma, stress, and adverse childhood experiences are associated with rapid weight gain in childhood and increased risk for adult obesity (S. E. Anderson et al., 2006; Santos et al., 2022). The COVID-19 pandemic has shone a particularly bright light on how stress and anxiety play a deleterious role in pediatric obesity and related outcomes (Alves et al., 2021; Wade et al., 2022). Such findings underscore the importance of addressing psychosocial factors in the treatment of pediatric obesity.

Suicidal Behaviors

Suicide is a leading cause of death in children, adolescents, and young adults (Hedegaard et al., 2021). Considering the bias, stigma, and social rejection associated with childhood obesity (Pont et al., 2017; Puhl & Lessard, 2020), researchers have explored the risk of increased suicidal behaviors among youth with excess weight. The findings are mixed. Data from the National Longitudinal Study of Adolescent to Adult Health showed no relationship between obesity and suicidal ideation in young adults (Graham & Frisco, 2022). Using another nationally representative data set, Zeller and colleagues (2013) found that weight status was associated with a significantly greater risk for suicidal ideation, but not suicide attempts. Given the rising prevalence of severe obesity in youth and the associated psychosocial pressures, clinicians working with this population should be equipped and prepared to assess and treat suicidality.

TREATMENT APPROACHES TO ADDRESS INTERNALIZING BEHAVIORS

The treatment of pediatric obesity typically entails lifestyle interventions that target dietary, physical activity, and sleep behaviors (Cadieux et al., 2016). Current recommendations for treatment indicate that effective pediatric weight management comprises interdisciplinary collaboration, including a behavioral health specialist such as a psychologist, counselor, or social worker (Hampl et al., 2023a). In addition to working with youth on motivation, goal setting, and adherence, behavioral health specialists are well suited to assess and treat internalizing behaviors that may be comorbid with pediatric obesity (Burton, Jones, et al., 2020).

Behavioral health specialists working with children and adolescents with obesity are encouraged to incorporate validated measures of psychosocial functioning in their assessment (Sagar & Gupta, 2018). For example, the Pediatric Symptom Checklist (PSC-17) is a brief screen that assesses internalizing (i.e., anxiety and depression), externalizing (i.e., disruptive behaviors and conduct problems), and attention difficulties as well as global psychosocial functioning (Murphy et al., 2016). Other options include the Strength and Difficulties Questionnaire (SDQ; R. Goodman, 1997), Child Behavior Checklist (CBCL; Achenbach & Edelbrock, 1991), Patient Health Questionnaire (PHQ-9 or PHQ-2; Kroenke et al., 2010), and Generalized Anxiety Disorder-7 (GAD-7; Spitzer et al., 2006).

There is strong evidence that addressing nutrition, exercise, and sleep hygiene is associated with improved psychosocial outcomes (Lassale et al., 2019; Walsh, 2011; X. Wang et al., 2022). For example, first-line treatment for mild to moderate depression includes scheduling physical activity and improving sleep hygiene (H. E. Brown et al., 2013; Davidson, 2010). Psychotherapy (e.g., cognitive behavior therapy [CBT], behavioral activation, interpersonal therapy) may be recommended as an alternative or an adjunct to medication.

Cognitive Behavior Therapy

CBT is a short-term, action-oriented, and problem-focused form of psychotherapy that focuses on how emotions and behaviors are influenced by maladaptive thought patterns (Craske, 2010). CBT uses several techniques to identify and change those patterns. Many of these techniques are applicable to weight management interventions as well as the treatment of internalizing behaviors. Several CBT techniques, along with practical treatment application examples, are listed in Table 11.1.

In a novel intervention to target symptoms of depression in adolescents with overweight and obesity, Jelalian and colleagues (2019) combined a CBT protocol that was modified to address healthy lifestyle behaviors with an exercise regimen. This intervention, termed *CBT plus healthy lifestyle*, enhances the CBT techniques of problem solving, cognitive restructuring, affect regulation, and behavioral activation to include attention to diet and physical activity. The intervention also includes psychoeducation on the relationship between depressed mood, weight, and physical activity. A trial of this program resulted in decreases in depressed mood and stabilization of weight. Interventions that address comorbid psychosocial and physical health problems are promising from efficacy and efficiency standpoints.

TABLE 11.1. Cognitive Behavioral Techniques

Technique	Description	Treatment application example
Goal setting	It is important to establish clear goals to help structure treatment and track progress. The SMART Goals Framework is used to help individuals articulate Specific, Measurable, Achievable, Realistic, and Time-based changes they want to see in their lives.	Darius is a 12-year-old boy who set a SMART Goal to increase his physical activity. He aimed to play soccer with his neighborhood league for 1 hour after school on Monday, Wednesday, and Thursday for the next 3 months.
Exposure	When incorporating lifestyle changes, youth and their families are often faced with new, unfamiliar, or previously avoided situations. Exposure encourages individuals to repeatedly face such situations to gradually increase their comfort and acceptance.	Jay is a 15-year-old who identifies as nonbinary. They have a strong dislike of green vegetables. In the beginning of treatment with a psychologist in a pediatric weight management program, Jay agrees to have one leaf of spinach on their plate; they do not have to eat the spinach. Over the course of 2 weeks, Jay progresses to smelling the spinach, touching the spinach to their tongue, taking a small bite of spinach that is spit out, and taking a small bite of spinach that is swallowed.
Problem solving	Effective problem solving involves helping an individual clearly define a problem, come up with various solutions, choose and implement the best solution, and evaluate the outcome to determine next steps. Problem solving emphasizes that problems are challenges to be solved rather than insurmountable obstacles.	Wanda's 4-year-old daughter, Lila, had a recent well-child visit during which the pediatrician encouraged healthier food choices because of concerns about rapid weight gain. Lila is cared for during the day by her paternal grandmother, who insists that it is her right to spoil Lila, and she provides Lila with candy, chips, and chocolate milk throughout the day. After thinking through several possible solutions to address this problem, Wanda decides that she could enroll Lila in a child care center or pack meals and snacks to accompany her daughter to the grandmother's house. She decides to try packing the meals and snacks for 1 month and then reevaluate whether Lila should be enrolled in a child care center.

(continues)

TABLE 11.1. Cognitive Behavioral Techniques (*Continued*)

Technique	Description	Treatment application example
Self-monitoring	Self-monitoring is a form of data gathering in which individuals observe and track targeted behaviors in order to monitor their progress or improvement over time.	Cornelius is a 16-year-old boy who is a candidate for bariatric surgery. He installs MyFitnessPal (https://www.myfitnesspal.com) on his phone to keep track of his daily water, protein, and fiber intake.
Stimulus control/ contingency management	It is important that individuals are aware of cues in their environment that encourage or discourage health behaviors. Stimulus control and contingency management involve changing environmental factors in ways that promote healthy lifestyle behaviors.	Daniel and Faye have three children. The family enjoys going on outings each weekend to spend time together. Daniel and Faye noticed that when they go to the local shopping mall for an outing, they tend to buy candy, popcorn, and fast food for everyone to eat. They realize that this is fine for an occasional treat but decide to limit trips to the mall to once every 2 months. On other weekends, they go to local parks and museums for their family outings.
Cognitive restructuring	Negative thoughts and beliefs can affect an individual's mood and behaviors. Cognitive restructuring is a technique for identifying automatic negative thoughts; challenging them; and ultimately replacing them with alternative, less distressing thoughts.	Lakshmi is an 8-year-old girl who was called fat and ugly by the other girls at a recent sleepover. She told her mother that every time she looks in the mirror, she remembers the mean comments and feels sad. Lakshmi's mother helps her come up with a list of positive attributes to rehearse every time she looks in a mirror. After practicing this for a few weeks, Lakshmi reports that when she looks in the mirror, her first thoughts are that she is beautiful, kind, and healthy.
Relapse prevention	Implementing change is difficult, and so is maintaining those changes. Relapse prevention is a strategy that helps individuals identify and avoid situations that are likely to get them off track in terms of healthy behaviors.	Darius, described in the first row of this table, set a SMART Goal to increase his physical activity through playing soccer with his neighborhood league. The season is coming to an end next week. In order to avoid going back to his routine of playing video games and snacking when he gets home from school, Darius talks with his parents about another activity he can engage in on Mondays, Wednesdays, and Thursdays. Together, they decide that Darius will begin tae kwon do lessons during the same timeframe once soccer season concludes.

Third-Wave Approaches

As CBT has grown and evolved over the years, new approaches have arisen that extend and expand traditional CBT to emphasize mindfulness, acceptance, and individual values and goals (S. C. Hayes & Hofmann, 2017). Treatments include acceptance and commitment therapy, dialectical behavior therapy, and mindfulness-based cognitive therapy. These third-wave approaches (see Chapter 5) have demonstrated interesting implications for the management of pediatric obesity and are discussed in more depth in Chapter 13.

Medications

The most commonly prescribed medications for pediatric internalizing behaviors are *selective serotonin reuptake inhibitors* (SSRIs). Practitioners tend to choose these medications because they are effective, nonaddictive, and have relatively few side effects (Locher et al., 2017). In addition to its effects on mood state, serotonin plays a role in appetite, food preference, and food intake (Reeves et al., 2008). The effect of SSRIs on available serotonin levels can potentially impede the body's metabolism of fat and sugar and can increase the desire for foods high in carbohydrates. It is important to note that SSRIs can take a while to work. Although some individuals may experience some symptom improvement within 1 to 2 weeks, it generally takes 4 to 6 weeks for the full benefit to be felt. SSRIs include fluoxetine (Prozac), paroxetine (Paxil), citalopram (Celexa), escitalopram (Lexapro), and sertraline (Zoloft). To date, however, fluoxetine is the only SSRI approved by the U.S. Food and Drug Administration for the treatment of depression in children and adolescents; escitalopram has been approved for use in adolescents. Sertraline, fluoxetine, and fluvoxamine (Luvox) are approved for treatment of obsessive-compulsive disorder in children. All other uses of SSRI to treat psychological functioning in children are considered off-label. Although serotonin norepinephrine reuptake inhibitors (SNRIs) have demonstrated efficacy in treatment of social anxiety, these medications should be considered as second- or third-line treatments because of limited trial data to support their use in pediatric populations (Garland et al., 2016).

Common side effects of SSRIs include agitation, nausea, gastrointestinal distress, insomnia, and changes to appetite. Research shows that SSRI use has been associated with weight loss in the short term but may be associated with weight gain with long-term use (S. H. Lee et al., 2016). Clinical studies suggest that some SNRIs (specifically, mirtazapine [Remeron]) and some tricyclic antidepressants (including amitriptyline [Elavil] and imipramine [Tofranil]) are also associated with weight gain.

OUTCOME OF THE CLINICAL CASE

At the initial evaluation, Charity expressed a strong desire to lose weight and improve her health; however, this strong desire was hampered by low motivation, which likely was due to her depressed mood. Despite her diagnosis of generalized anxiety disorder, it seems that many of Charity's fears revolved around negative evaluation and judgments. At the conclusion of the intake, the clinician provided psychoeducation on the importance of medication adherence and highlighted that the type of medication Charity was being prescribed must build up in her system before she will feel the full benefit. The clinician also emphasized the importance of having open and honest conversations with her psychiatrist about how her medication makes her feel.

Adolescents often feel invulnerable to the risks associated with their health behaviors. In Charity's case, it seems that her symptoms of anxiety and amotivation were impeding her ability to adhere to medical recommendations, thereby negatively affecting her obesity and endocrinological conditions. Understanding the limits of her motivation, as well as being aware of behaviors such as secretive eating, were key to developing an efficacious treatment plan.

Another key was sensitive navigation of the role of her parents in treatment. Children and adolescents have limited control over their environment, and as they mature, youth tend to seek more autonomy. Because Charity's parents are separated, it is likely that rules regarding eating, exercise, and sleep regimen differ across households. Charity expressed frustration over her mother's food choices and irritation at her parents' attempts to influence her health behaviors, and this defiance seemed to hinder the uptake of desired health behaviors. As such, it was important to focus on supporting Charity in implementing behavior changes more independently by helping her understand her personal motivations and readiness to change.

At subsequent follow-up sessions in the pediatric weight management clinic, Charity engaged in behavioral activation and goal setting by scheduling a 15-minute walk each day after school. She reports that in the beginning, it was difficult to take a walk every day, but after following the schedule she set for herself she started to feel more confident and noticed that she was actually looking forward to her walks. She also reports that walking every day inspired her to return to the gym; she replaced 2 days of walking with workouts at the gym. Using stimulus control, Charity keeps her gym bag in the passenger seat of her car so that she is prompted to head to the gym as soon as she gets out of school.

CONCLUSION

The strong associations between pediatric obesity and internalizing behaviors merit additional attention in the assessment and treatment of youth presenting with excess weight. Behavioral health specialists working in the context of pediatric weight management play an important role in supporting not only youth with clinical levels of internalizing behaviors, but also children and adolescents who endorse subclinical sadness, worries, or low self-esteem. Preventive support may lead to better mental and physical health outcomes.

KEY POINTS

- Pediatric obesity can be both a cause and consequence of internalizing behavior concerns.

- Many evidence-based treatments can be modified to address co-occurring internalizing behaviors and pediatric obesity.

THINKING OUTSIDE THE BOX

Given the cyclical nature of obesity and internalizing behaviors, what factors influence which symptoms should be prioritized for treatment?

12

EXTERNALIZING SYMPTOMS AND DISORDERS

CLINICAL CASE INTRODUCTION

David is an 8-year-old non-Hispanic Black male who presented to an out-patient interdisciplinary pediatric obesity clinic with his mother and grand-mother for health and behavior intervention at the recommendation of his pediatrician because of his weight gain. David's body mass index at the initial psychological visit in the clinic was 41.4, which is above the 99th percentile for his age and sex and falls in the Class 3, or severe obesity, range. His family reports that David's weight gain had been normal until he was about 4 years old, when his grandfather passed away. Developmentally, he was born about 1 month early and weighed 7 lbs, 3 oz (~3 kg). After birth, he spent a few days in the neonatal intensive care unit because of pneumonia. His family reports that David reached normal developmental milestones, and he did not have a history of receiving speech, occupational, or physical therapy or of feeding- or eating-related concerns. David currently lives with his maternal

(continues)

https://doi.org/10.1037/0000401-012
Psychological Approaches to the Treatment of Pediatric Obesity, by C. S. Lim and E. T. Burton

CLINICAL CASE INTRODUCTION (Continued)

grandmother, mother, and older sister. David's parents are reportedly still married, but his father lives elsewhere and has limited involvement in his life. David reports seeing his father about every 1 to 2 months.

David's family reports significant financial concerns. David recently finished second grade and is advancing to third grade at a public school. His family denies he has issues with learning and claims he received all As during the school year. However, they do report issues with his behavior at school. They report that his behavior ratings throughout the school year were mostly unacceptable (red on the behavior rating scale) because of difficulty completing classwork and homework. David was suspended two times during the previous school year because of behavioral issues. Socially, his family reports that he is liked by most kids his age, but he has experienced bullying from older kids who ride his bus. David reports having one friend. He is not involved in extracurricular activities. He spends a lot of time playing on his computer and listening to music.

With regard to eating, his family reports that David says he is hungry all the time and begs them often for food, even after eating meals. He generally eats three meals and one snack per day, but he has trouble controlling portion sizes and gets angry when his family tries to help him choose healthier foods, or smaller portions to eat. David's grandmother reports that he eats few vegetables but does consume a variety of fruits. According to his family, he initially did well making changes to his eating habits for a short time, but the changes are hard for him to maintain. His grandmother expresses concern regarding David sneaking food and sugary drinks.

For physical activity, David has tried playing active video games. He reports not liking to go outside, and his family states that he often refuses to engage in physical activity. Specific to behavioral and emotional functioning, David's family expresses concerns regarding his behavior at home. He physically fights with his older sister, which often occurs when she refuses to play with him. They indicate that it is a struggle to get him to complete his chores, and he curses and threatens to hit his mother. They also describe him as deliberately annoying family members, and when he gets angry he destroys toys and other objects.

David has been prescribed multiple psychiatric medications (lisdexamfetamine dimesylate [Vyvanse] and clonidine [Catapres]) to manage his behavior by a provider at a local community mental health center. He has also received some counseling services at the community mental health center, but the family describes difficulties related to receiving consistent counseling services. He does not have a history of inpatient psychiatric hospitalization.

BEHAVIORAL AND EXTERNALIZING SYMPTOMS APPLICABLE TO PEDIATRIC OBESITY

During childhood, externalizing and behavioral symptoms, such as inattention, hyperactivity, and impulsivity, are common (Mechler et al., 2022). Oppositionality is also common and developmentally normative in early childhood (American Psychiatric Association, 2022). Externalizing behaviors are influenced by cognitive abilities, such as executive functioning and self-regulation skills, as well as other factors related to social, emotional, and language development (Kremer et al., 2016). Children also commonly display behavioral symptoms in the context of feeding and eating and physical activity, which affect prevention and treatment efforts made by psychologists and other health care providers to address pediatric obesity. For example, being able to sit at the table for the duration of a family meal may influence the amount of vegetables a child eats; similarly, a child's refusal to play basketball outside affects their engagement in physical activity. Understanding the role of executive functioning and self-regulation skills, and recognizing normative externalizing symptoms, as well as those that may be more severe and require additional consideration and treatment, are important for psychologists and other behavioral health specialists involved in developing pediatric obesity prevention and treatment efforts.

EXECUTIVE FUNCTIONING AND SELF-REGULATION

There is a body of research that has examined associations between executive functioning and self-regulation and obesity that has specifically focused on whether and how poorer executive functioning and self-regulation skills increase obesity risk. *Executive functioning* is recognized as higher level cognitive functioning, such as planning, organizing, and problem solving (Gowey et al., 2021), and it develops throughout childhood and adolescence (V. Anderson et al., 2008). Goal-directed behavior is considered the result of executive functioning skills and involves specific domains such as working memory, inhibition, and monitoring (Gutierrez-Colina et al., 2022). Some scholars have speculated that poorer executive functioning skills may lead to engagement in unhealthy eating behaviors, which then leads to weight gain (La Marra et al., 2022). Previous research with adults and youth has examined associations between executive functioning and weight status. Cross-sectional studies have typically found significant differences in executive functioning between individuals with obesity and those without obesity

(Favieri et al., 2019). One study that compared five different domains of executive functioning in adults with overweight and obesity found significant group differences only in working memory (Sánchez-SanSegundo et al., 2021).

Another study that compared adults with overweight/obesity with adults who were not overweight found no significant group differences in executive functioning when sex, age, and education level were controlled (La Marra et al., 2022). These results suggest the complex role sociodemographic characteristics play in associations between cognitive skills, such as executive functioning, and obesity risk. In youth with obesity, those with poorer executive functioning skills are more likely to engage in disordered eating behaviors (Gowey et al., 2018), and as the severity of executive functioning impairments increases so does engagement in more overeating and binge eating behaviors, as do symptoms of behavioral problems (Gowey et al., 2020).

There has been interest in examining potential mechanisms that may explain the association between executive functioning and weight in youth. Genetic links between weight and executive functioning have been found, with one study estimating that genetic influences account for approximately 80% of the association (Wood et al., 2019). Preliminary research has also focused on inflammation and revealed that greater adiposity in youth is associated with greater inflammation, which is then associated with reduced executive functioning skills (King et al., 2023). However, this evidence is from cross-sectional research with small sample sizes; more research focused on potential mechanisms that explain this association is needed.

An additional area of research that has examined associations between executive functioning and weight status is related to response to weight management interventions. There is some evidence that poorer executive functioning skills in children and adults lead to worse response to weight management interventions but that interventions designed specifically to improve executive functioning have not led to weight loss (Du et al., 2021). More research is needed to determine the potential role that improved executive functioning skills may play in pediatric weight management prevention and treatment efforts.

Executive functioning is also thought to be related to self-regulation skills in a variety of emotional and behavioral contexts, including engagement and management of health-related behaviors. Broadly, *self-regulation* has been identified as the ability to manage emotions, behaviors, attention, and cognition (Gagne et al., 2021). In early childhood, self-regulation skills specific to the eating context have been cross-sectionally associated with weight status, but associations between general executive functioning and weight status have not been found (S. O. Hughes et al., 2015). However, longitudinal research has found evidence that early self-regulation skills predict weight status when children were both 3 and 8 years older than at the time self-regulation skills were initially assessed (Graziano et al., 2010, 2013).

In summary, although research findings are mixed, and more work is needed to understand potential mechanisms, executive functioning and self-regulation skills are important for psychologists and health care professionals to consider in the context of pediatric obesity prevention and treatment. Executive functioning and self-regulation skills are typically impaired when youth exhibit significant externalizing symptoms or are diagnosed with an externalizing disorder.

EXTERNALIZING DISORDERS

In general, the presence of comorbid externalizing disorders, such as attention-deficit/hyperactivity disorder (ADHD), oppositional defiant disorder (ODD), and conduct disorder (CD), are important to consider in the prevention and treatment of pediatric obesity. Externalizing disorders are diagnosed in approximately 10% of children and adolescents (X. Wu et al., 2018) and are the most common reason youth are referred to mental health services (Riise et al., 2021). Thus, psychologists and other mental health providers working in the area of pediatric obesity are likely to treat children and families experiencing both externalizing issues and overweight and obesity concerns. Specific externalizing disorders and research findings unique to pediatric obesity prevention and treatment are reviewed in the sections that follow.

Attention-Deficit/Hyperactivity Disorder

The prevalence of ADHD in youth in the United States is estimated to be approximately 8% (Bozinovic et al., 2021), and similar rates have been found worldwide (Mechler et al., 2022). ADHD affects functioning in a variety of domains (e.g., behavioral, social, emotional, academic) and entails a significant cost to both the health care and educational systems. For example, the societal cost of ADHD has been estimated to be over $120 million annually in the United States (Zhao et al., 2019). There is increasing evidence that ADHD is associated with an increased risk of overweight and obesity. Children and adults with ADHD are more likely to have overweight or obesity compared with those without ADHD (Cortese et al., 2016). Children with ADHD and poor executive functioning skills are at additional risk for overweight and obesity (Graziano et al., 2012). Rates of ADHD in samples of children with obesity in the United States range from 10% to 17.6% (Merrill et al., 2021), which are higher than national estimates in the general pediatric population. Theoretical hypotheses to explain associations between ADHD symptoms and obesity risk include impulsivity and inattention (hallmark symptoms of ADHD) as being risk factors for later weight gain. In addition, youth with both ADHD and obesity often have reward deficit syndromes, such as impaired delay gratification; also, insufficient dopamine levels are a characteristic of both ADHD and obesity (Cuda et al., 2022). ADHD symptoms are positively associated with disordered eating behaviors in youth with overweight and obesity (Gowey et al., 2017), which could also explain the association. Specific ADHD symptoms, such as difficulties with attention and planning, may result in skipped meals as well as decreased engagement in physical activity (Cuda et al., 2022). Likewise, impulsivity may result in binge eating behaviors.

Inflammation is another mechanism that has been evaluated in the literature as potentially linking obesity and ADHD in youth. For example, Cortese and colleagues (2019) found that increased inflammation levels (assessed from bloodwork) were associated with increased severity of ADHD symptoms in youth ages 6 to 18 years . However, this was a pilot study, and the authors described a need for both larger, and longitudinal, studies to further explore inflammation as a potential mechanism to explain the associations between ADHD and obesity.

Intensive lifestyle-based weight management treatments often involve organization, planning, and attentional control, which are hallmark deficits in ADHD. ADHD symptoms in adults have been linked to limited treatment response to intensive weight management interventions (Cortese & Castellanos, 2014). Similar patterns have been discovered in randomized clinical trials examining pediatric obesity interventions, even those that primarily examined parenting-focused interventions targeting young children (Eiffener et al., 2019). Thus, assessing the presence and severity of ADHD symptoms is important in pediatric obesity prevention and treatment settings.

Oppositional Defiant Disorder and Conduct Disorder

ODD and CD have substantial global health burdens in terms of social, economic, and education costs (Nujić et al., 2021). Although research that has examined associations between ODD and CD and pediatric obesity is more sparse than research on ADHD and obesity, there is evidence of increased prevalence of both ODD and CD in children with obesity compared with children without obesity (Nujić et al., 2021; Smith & Mason, 2022). For example, children with obesity are 30% more likely to have ODD than children without obesity (Smith & Mason, 2022). The results of a meta-analysis revealed a 32% increased risk of CD in children with overweight and obesity (Nujić et al., 2021). Taken together, these studies suggest that behavioral problems are likely present before weight gain and predict future weight gain (Matheson & Eichen, 2018). Inflammation has also been linked to conduct problems, which may be one potential explanation regarding comorbidities between obesity and ODD and CD, but more research is needed to further explore these associations (Cortese et al., 2019). Associations between weight status and externalizing disorders in youth are also influenced by medications.

MEDICATIONS FOR EXTERNALIZING DISORDERS

In the context of the prevention and treatment of pediatric obesity, it is also important for mental health providers to be aware that any medications children have been or are currently prescribed to treat externalizing symptoms could influence weight status in a variety of ways. For example, some medications may affect appetite, whereas others may change metabolism and other biological characteristics that may lead to weight-related changes.

Clinical guidelines for the treatment of ADHD emphasize medication as part of the treatment approach (Mechler et al., 2022), which is determined in part on the basis of the severity of symptoms and the medication's impact on functioning in academic and psychosocial settings. Stimulant medications, such as methylphenidate (e.g., Ritalin, Concerta) and lisdexamfetamine dimesylate (Vyvanse), are commonly considered the first line of medical treatment for ADHD and are prescribed to youth by a variety of medical providers in primary care and specialty care medical settings. Lisdexamfetamine dimesylate is a stimulant medication approved by the U.S. Food and Drug Administration that is used to treat ADHD in children ages 6 years and older and for adults with binge eating disorder.

Children with comorbid obesity and ADHD may be prescribed lisdexamfetamine dimesylate (on- or off-label) to help with symptoms associated with binge eating and loss-of-control eating (V. R. Johnson et al., 2020). Common side effects of stimulant medications include decreased appetite and reduced body mass index because of potential weight loss. There are some concerns related to the potential for symptoms to rebound when medication effects wear off in the afternoon and evening hours, which may affect appetite and eating behavior or potentially result in binge eating behavior. This issue has previously been discussed in the context of family-based pediatric obesity treatment (C. S. Lim et al., 2014). Stimulant medications are now available in both short- and long-acting formulations, so if rebound effects are present then exploring the utility of switching to a long-acting medication would be important. Adding an additional short-term dose of the medication later in the day could also be considered. Nonstimulant medications, such as atomoxetine (Strattera), clonidine (Catapres), and guanfacine (Tenex, Intuniv), are typically considered second-line treatments for ADHD (Mechler et al., 2022). Side effects associated with these medications include decreased appetite, sleep issues, fatigue, and sedation, all of which may influence engagement in healthy lifestyle behaviors such as eating and physical activity.

For children with ODD or CD, the nonstimulant medications just mentioned may be prescribed to address behavioral symptoms. In addition, atypical or second-generation antipsychotics, such as risperidone (Risperdal), are commonly prescribed to treat severe behavioral disorders that may or may not be associated with intellectual disability and/or autism spectrum disorders (Reekie et al., 2015). Weight gain is a common side effect associated with these medications, and systematic reviews have indicated that they can result in clinically significant weight gain in children and adolescents; thus, the dose and length of treatment are important factors to consider.

Although increased appetite is largely attributed to increases in weight as a result of these medications, there is some evidence that atypical antipsychotic medications may affect metabolism and decrease energy expenditure associated with physical activity (Reekie et al., 2015). Adding a medication to counteract the weight gain side effects of antipsychotic medications may also be helpful for prescribing providers to consider on the basis of the available research. Although more research is needed to confirm this finding, supplementing treatment to counteract weigh gain side effects, especially if weight concerns are already present, may be an option. The effectiveness of weight management treatments could be affected while patients are taking various psychiatric medications, and it is important to communicate this to patients, their families, and treatment teams.

For children with comorbid obesity and externalizing disorders, it is vital for there to be collaboration among the prescribing provider, psychiatrists, pharmacists, and psychologists or mental health care providers to ensure that appropriate medical and psychological treatments do not impede either the potential success of weight management prevention and treatment efforts or the effectiveness of prescribed medications. It is important for psychological providers to be aware of psychiatric medications that can promote or reduce weight gain and be comfortable providing families with education and problem-solving strategies to address these potential concerns. Psychologists should also assess adherence to medications prescribed for child behavioral concerns and intervene with families if needed. Referring patients to or consulting with other medical providers about potential medication side effects, and discussing other medications that may help balance the treatment of the behavioral issues and the prevention or treatment of weight concerns, also is important.

EVIDENCE-BASED PSYCHOLOGICAL TREATMENTS TO CONSIDER

For mental health providers working in pediatric obesity prevention and treatment settings, identifying evidence-based treatments that can be used to address childhood behavior problems and health behaviors is important. In general, there are decades of research evidence demonstrating the efficacy of parenting interventions in improving both parent–child relationships and child behaviors, and they are considered the gold standard for treating externalizing disorders in youth (Kong et al., 2023). Positive parenting interventions reduce the risk of overweight/obesity in children even when they do not focus specifically on changing health behaviors (e.g., eating, physical activity). Specific evidence-based parenting interventions have also been adapted to prevent and treat pediatric obesity. For example, a form of parent–child interaction therapy (PCIT) has been developed, called *PCIT-Health*, to decrease pediatric obesity risk in young children at high risk (Domoff & Niec, 2018). The adapted treatment includes traditional Child-Directed Interactions and Parent-Directed Interactions of PCIT but also includes an added Health-Directed Interaction component that focuses on parenting feeding style and parenting related to screen time use.

Parenting skills have also been integrated into pediatric obesity treatment programs for youth at various ages. A pediatric obesity treatment for children ages 2 to 5 years that was conducted in both clinical and home settings incorporated child behavioral management skills, which focused on praise and attention to increase healthy eating and physical activity; ignoring and time-outs to deal with tantrums; contingency management; modeling; and stimulus control (Stark et al., 2011). Compared with youth and caregivers who received standard care, those who participated in a parenting skills program had better weight outcomes 6 and 12 months after treatment. Behavioral parenting skills have also been incorporated into numerous weight management programs for children and adolescents and overall have demonstrated small treatment effects (Janicke et al., 2014).

Intensive summer treatment programs are supported by a large body of research demonstrating their effectiveness at improving ADHD symptoms in youth (Fabiano et al., 2014). These programs incorporate parenting skills training so that the behavioral modification system used in the summer program will transfer to the home environment. There has been an interest in modifying summer treatment programs, given their inclusion of sports and physical activity, to address pediatric overweight and obesity, and pilot results have been promising (Graziano et al., 2017). Given that there is strong evidence from the fields of child externalizing disorders and pediatric weight management, behavioral parenting interventions may be the first-line psychological treatment strategy to implement if a child has comorbid obesity and externalizing behavioral problems. However, the setting (clinic, community, home, school, virtual, etc.), format (caregiver only, caregiver and child), and structure of the parenting intervention can vary and be individualized according to patient, family, and community characteristics.

Cognitive behavior therapy (CBT) has also been implemented with children and adolescents (N. R. Kang & Kwack, 2020). CBT for pediatric obesity focuses on behavioral strategies to change eating and physical activity behaviors through monitoring and cognitive components to address distorted body image and expand emotion-regulation skills. Recent work has demonstrated improvements in both weight and ADHD symptoms when they are targeted in CBT. CBT has been identified as being an important treatment approach with individuals who have comorbid psychiatric concerns in the context of interdisciplinary pediatric obesity treatment; thus, it should be considered by psychologists and other mental health providers in the context of pediatric obesity prevention and treatment efforts.

OUTCOME OF THE CLINICAL CASE

At the initial evaluation, David was diagnosed with ADHD and ODD, and the following four recommendations were provided to the family. First, cognitive behavioral and parenting-focused psychological therapy were suggested to address behavioral concerns as well as engagement in healthy lifestyle behaviors. The family expressed concerns, however, about receiving regular psychological services in the clinic because they lived about 1 hour away. They were interested in being seen frequently by a provider in their community and scheduling follow-up psychological appointments in the weight management clinic about once a month. Second, for treatment in the community, David was referred to a community-based comprehensive child

OUTCOME OF THE CLINICAL CASE (*Continued*)

mental health facility that provides individual and parenting/family therapy in both the school and home settings. Third, David and his family were encouraged to continue attending follow-up psychiatry appointments at his local community mental health center for the medication management of his behavioral symptoms. Last, David's mother and grandmother were provided with general behavioral parenting recommendations regarding strategies to help improve behavioral adherence for children with attention and behavioral problems that could also be applied to healthy lifestyle behaviors (see Table 12.1 and Exhibits 12.1–12.4).

After the initial visit, David and his family no-showed to multiple follow-up appointments with medical and psychological providers in the clinic (attrition rates in pediatric weight management clinics are approximately 45%; Morrow et al., 2020). A couple of years after David was lost to follow-up, the team learned that David had ended up hospitalized on a child psychiatric inpatient unit because of increasing behavioral problems and suicidal ideation. During this time, he had continued to gain weight, and his body mass index increased significantly. At the time of admission to the pediatric psychiatry unit, he was living with his grandmother and siblings after having spent time in foster care. During his inpatient psychiatric hospitalization, the psychiatry providers consulted with members of the pediatric weight management team because of concerns regarding David being overly focused on food, as well as his continued weight gain and related health complications. A recommendation was made that nutrition services be integrated into David's inpatient treatment. Nutrition professionals provided recommendations regarding how to restrict his caloric intake. David mostly responded well to nutrition changes, but after a couple of weeks he started to complain about wanting more food. The psychiatry team explained the need for dietary recommendations to him, and his complaints decreased. David spent another week in the hospital and was discharged after his behavior improved.

After his discharge, David continued to receive counseling and psychiatric services in the community, but there continued to be an escalation of behavioral problems, and he was again hospitalized in a pediatric inpatient psychiatric facility. David was eventually transferred to a child residential psychiatric facility for long-term medical and psychotherapy treatment because his grandmother felt like she was not able to manage his behaviors. David agreed to receive residential treatment because he felt like he needed more help. While living in the residential facility, he was seen at

(continues)

OUTCOME OF THE CLINICAL CASE *(Continued)*

the pediatric weight management clinic for follow-up. David reported that the prepared meals and snacks at the residential facility helped by controlling his access to types of food and portion sizes. The facility also integrated regular exercise into his daily routine, which was available through a playground and other resources at the facility. David reported that he had started to enjoy exercising regularly. At the residential facility, David reported learning coping skills to manage his anger and frustration, such as reading and going outside. He was also treated with psychotropic medications, specifically, methylphenidate (Ritalin) for management of ADHD symptoms and trazodone (e.g., Desyrel, Oleptro) for sleep-related issues. David planned to return to live with his grandmother after he completed residential treatment. His treatment plan included outpatient counseling and psychiatry services through the community-based mental health setting and continued follow-up clinic visits with the pediatric weight management team for monitoring and assessment, as well as for additional support for him and his family regarding the continued implementation of lifestyle changes at home.

TABLE 12.1. Example of Adapted Behavioral Parenting Skills Handouts Focused on Healthy Lifestyle Behaviors

Encouraging and Supporting Your Child: PRIDE Skills for Healthy Lifestyle Behaviors		
Skills	**Reasons**	**Examples**
Praise appropriate behavior	• Increases the likelihood that your child's good behavior will increase. • Lets your child know you like and notice their behaviors.	• Child behavior: Child takes a bite of his or her carrot sticks at snack time. • Caregiver response: "Good job trying the carrots for snack!"
Reinforce appropriate behavior with nonverbals	• Nonverbals can also send powerful messages to your child about what behavior is appropriate. • Nonverbals should be used in combination with Praise (especially when beginning to make healthy lifestyle changes).	• Child behavior: Child takes a drink of water. • Caregiver response: (Gives child a high-five) "I really like how you took a drink of water."
Imitate appropriate table behavior	• Shows your child that you like his or her behavior. • Increases your child's self-esteem.	• Child behavior: Child puts a raisin on his or her celery. • Caregiver response: Puts a raisin on their celery.
Describe appropriate behavior	• Shows your child that you are interested in what he or she is doing. • Can be more effective when used in combination with imitation.	• Child Behavior: Child uses a napkin. • Caregiver response: (Cleans own face with a napkin) "You used your napkin to keep your face clean. That's a good idea."
Be Enthusiastic	• Increases positive interactions between you and your child.	• Child behavior: Child puts cup on kitchen counter after dinner. • Caregiver response: "Thank you for being such a GREAT helper by putting your cup on the counter!"

Note. Information in this table was adapted from various materials, including Eyberg and Funderburk (2011), Janicke et al. (2011), and Hembree-Kigin and McNeil (1995).

EXHIBIT 12.1. Positive Attention for Appropriate Behavior

Attending means paying attention to your child when they are behaving appropriately. Positive attention helps children feel good about themselves—and a positive view of themselves is important when they are beginning to make changes to their health behaviors.

Ways to provide positive attention and attend to your child's appropriate behavior:

1. Praise
2. Describing their appropriate behavior
3. Physical touch (e.g., high-fives, pats on the back)
4. Smiling (and other nonverbals, e.g., thumbs-up)
5. Rewards or special privileges
6. Spending time with your child

Rules for effective praise and attention

Rule 1: Be immediate. This helps kids remember to repeat good behavior. Catch them being good right away!

Rule 2: Be consistent. For example, every time they choose a fruit at breakfast provide them with praise or other types of positive attention.

Rule 3: Praise often! This is especially important when families start working on making healthy lifestyle changes. Lots of support and encouragement are crucial!

Rule 4: Be specific, and keep comments brief. Example: "I am proud of you for choosing a vegetable for your snack!" Describe the specific behavior you are praising.

Note. Information in this exhibit was adapted from various materials, including Eyberg and Funderburk (2011), Janicke et al. (2011), and Hembree-Kigin and McNeil (1995).

EXHIBIT 12.2. Motivating and Supporting Your Child

Differential attention means ignoring inappropriate behavior. Your attention is a powerful tool. Positive attention can be used to reinforce appropriate behavior, while ignoring can be used to decrease attention seeking behavior like whining, complaining, or temper tantrums.

Guidelines for using ignoring

- Choose behaviors that you are confident you can ignore (e.g., complaints about not getting a dessert after dinner).
- Refrain from any verbal or nonverbal attention (no frowning, sighing, scolding, or "mom" looks).
- Once you start ignoring a behavior, like a tantrum, continue to ignore until the behavior stops.
- Use together with praise for appropriate behavior. Immediately provide praise for appropriate behavior (e.g., using a calm voice).
  - Consistently ignore the inappropriate behavior. As children realize that this behavior will no longer get them what they want, the behavior will eventually decrease.
  - Be prepared for the behavior to increase in frequency or intensity when initially starting to use ignoring (this is called an *extinction burst*) and continue to ignore until the behavior decreases in frequency or intensity.
- Provide praise for siblings, other children, or adults who are engaging in the behavior you want to see out of the target child.

More must-haves for dealing with resistance

- Give choices. Example: "Would you like an apple or a banana for a snack?"
- Set clear expectations and make the rules in advance. Example: "You have to pick at least one vegetable to put on your sandwich."
- Refer to consequences and follow through.
- Pick your battles.
- Be consistent.
- Do not expect perfection.
- Maintain a sense of humor.

Note. Information in this exhibit was adapted from various materials, including Eyberg and Funderburk (2011), Janicke et al. (2011), and Hembree-Kigin and McNeil (1995).

EXHIBIT 12.3. Giving Effective Commands to Encourage Healthy Habits

As you continue to encourage healthy habits in your child, you will also be giving your child more directives to try new things, such as new foods, less preferred foods, and new family routines.

- Get everyone one the same page by giving effective commands.
  - Commands are directives/instructions that make it clear that you expect your child to do a certain behavior. example: "Take a sip of your milk, please."
- Commands can be used to shape behaviors, such as learning to taste and eat healthier foods. However, commands should be used sparingly.
  - Too many commands can be frustrating to children and teens.
  - Too many commands decrease the frequency of your positive attention.
  - Use commands to help shape *specific* behaviors that you feel are important.
  - For less important behaviors, rather than a command, allow your child to have choices. Example: "Would you like to have cucumbers or carrots for your vegetable?" This gives your child a choice between two healthy vegetables.

Note. Information in this exhibit was adapted from various materials, including Eyberg and Funderburk (2011), Janicke et al. (2011), and Hembree-Kigin and McNeil (1995).

EXHIBIT 12.4. Tips for Giving Effective Commands

- Commands should be explained before they are given or after your child complies.
  - Explaining the reasons for your commands teaches your child about social rules and helps shape a predictable environment.
- Make the command a statement (direct command), not a question.
  - Make sure your child understands that you are giving them instructions that you expect to be followed.
  - Statements make it clear that your request is an expectation and not a choice. Example: "Take one sip of your water."
  - Questions imply choice and give your child the option to say "No"! Example: "Could you please take one sip of your water?"
- Describe the specific positive behavior you expect.
  - Describing the positive behavior makes your expectation of your child clear. Example: "Take one sip of your water."
  - Describing the negative behaviors, only communicates what you don't want them to do. Example: "Stop asking for juice."
  - Vague commands can be confusing and result in your child getting in trouble, not because they weren't being mindful but because they didn't understand. Example: "Put it down."
- Make sure you have their attention.
  - Begin a command by saying your child's name to ensure that they know that you are talking to them.
  - Pause briefly before giving your command to give your child time to shift their attention to you.

EXHIBIT 12.4. Tips for Giving Effective Commands (*Continued*)

- Use the 5-second rule to allow your child time to comply. If they don't comply, give them a warning about the consequence. Example: "If you do not take a taste, you will not get a sticker."
- Give one command at a time.
  - Children, especially those who are younger or have known attention problems, generally have short attention spans and will have difficulty remembering more than one request/instruction.
  - Break multistep commands into individual commands that are given one at a time and, when followed, individually praised.
- Stay calm when making requests.
  - Use a calm but matter-of-fact tone to help communicate the importance of your request.
  - Yelling teaches children that they need to comply with your requests only when you are angry.
- Give a command only if you are prepared to follow through.
  - Know what the age-appropriate consequence will be for complying. Examples: specific verbal praise ("Good job tasting your snack!"), a high-five, a sticker.
  - Know what the age-appropriate consequence will be for not complying. Examples: child does not get a high-five, verbal praise, sticker.
  - If you are not prepared to follow through with a consequence, do not give a command.

Note. Information in this exhibit was adapted from various materials, including Eyberg and Funderburk (2011), Janicke et al. (2011), and Hembree-Kigin and McNeil (1995).

CONCLUSION

Executive functioning and self-regulation skills, as well as the presence of externalizing symptoms and disorders, are important to screen and integrate into pediatric obesity prevention and treatment programs. To better understand the potential role medication plays with regard to weight gain or difficulties achieving weight loss, as well as with regard to medications that may help with both medical/health and behavioral concerns, psychologists working with youth with comorbid deficits in executive functioning, self-regulation skills, and/or externalizing behavioral problems and obesity would benefit from collaborating and consulting with medical and mental health care providers who prescribe psychiatric medications (e.g., pediatricians, medical providers in weight management centers, psychiatrists, or psychiatric nurse practitioners). Many components of psychological evidence-based treatments for childhood externalizing symptoms and disorders have and can be modified to address healthy lifestyle behaviors, specifically, eating and physical activity, as well as other health behaviors associated with pediatric obesity prevention and treatment.

KEY POINTS

- Pediatric obesity prevention and treatment strategies should take into account executive functioning, self-regulation, and externalizing symptoms and disorders.

- Parenting programs and other empirically supported interventions for externalizing symptoms can be modified to include health behaviors.

THINKING OUTSIDE THE BOX

How does systematic racism influence the presentation of comorbid externalizing symptoms and obesity in youth?

13

DISORDERED EATING BEHAVIORS

CLINICAL CASE INTRODUCTION

Prentice is a 15-year-old non-Hispanic White male who presented to an out-patient interdisciplinary pediatric weight management clinic with a history of Blount disease, which was diagnosed at age 13 years. His body mass index (BMI) at this visit was 56.54, which is greater than the 99th percentile for his age and sex and is classified as Class 3, or severe obesity. He has significant bowing in his left leg and complains of pain when walking. He also has diagnoses of type 2 diabetes and severe obstructive sleep apnea. He was referred by orthopedic specialists and has been recommended for osteotomy, a surgery to realign the bones in his leg. However, because of the severity of his obesity, the surgical team is hesitant to proceed until he loses a significant amount of weight.

(continues)

https://doi.org/10.1037/0000401-013
Psychological Approaches to the Treatment of Pediatric Obesity, by C. S. Lim and E. T. Burton

CLINICAL CASE INTRODUCTION *(Continued)*

During his initial psychological evaluation with the weight management clinic, Prentice reports a moderately strong desire to lose weight (8 out of 10). His mother reports that her son has always carried extra weight and looks just like the other men in the family. She recounts multiple attempts over the years at losing weight, stating that they have tried every diet and exercise plan she could find in magazines, on TV, or online. Prentice expresses frustration that nothing he tried has ever worked. He endorses engaging in loss-of-control eating multiple times per month and states that he typically seeks food when stressed, bored, or lonely.

Prentice shares that he is angry and frustrated with his life circumstances. He reports that he is attending high school virtually because he can no longer walk the distances between classes. His mother states that Prentice is often subjected to cruel comments about his weight and limp; she says that a desire to limit this negative attention also factored into the decision to have Prentice attend school virtually. Prentice reports that he has few friends and often feels lonely. His social isolation and accompanying negative emotion contribute to a cycle of binge eating to cope with emotional distress, which in turn exacerbates his obesity and impedes his candidacy for an osteotomy. Prentice says he feels it is unfair that he needs to lose weight in order to be eligible to have a surgery that could improve his life.

DISORDERED EATING BEHAVIORS

Approximately 30 million individuals in the United States experience symptoms of disordered eating (Galmiche et al., 2019; Hudson et al., 2007; Le Grange et al., 2012). Eating disorders (e.g., anorexia nervosa [AN], bulimia nervosa [BN], and binge eating disorder [BED]) are especially prevalent among adolescents (Swanson et al., 2011).[1] Considering the associated consequences, such as impaired quality of life, increased health care costs, and high mortality rates, disordered eating among adolescents signifies a major

---

[1] Whereas the term *eating disorder* indicates a clinical diagnosis, *disordered eating* refers to abnormal eating patterns that, taken alone, do not meet diagnostic criteria. An individual with an eating disorder may exhibit disordered eating behaviors, but not all individuals engaging in disordered eating will be diagnosed with an eating disorder.

public health concern (Ward et al., 2019). BED is of particular concern given that its lifetime prevalence rates exceed those of AN and BN combined (Hudson et al., 2007; National Institute of Mental Health, 2016). It is the most common eating disorder.

The co-occurrence of eating disorders and pediatric obesity is not well understood, although many clinical and community studies to date have demonstrated that obesity and eating disorders can coexist. A strong association between obesity and disordered eating, in particular, BED, has been identified in adults and adolescents (Duncan et al., 2017; J. F. Hayes et al., 2018). The heightened risk of medical, psychological, and social sequelae make adolescents experiencing obesity and disordered eating especially vulnerable (Jebeile et al., 2021). Despite the intersecting health risks, some clinicians and researchers have argued that efforts to prevent or treat pediatric obesity through dietary change or energy restriction can inadvertently elicit body dissatisfaction, unhealthy weight control patterns, and binge eating behaviors (Lebow, Sim, et al., 2015; Neumark-Sztainer, 2009; Sim et al., 2013). However, a recent systematic review and meta-analysis reported that structured and well-run pediatric obesity treatment was associated with short- and long-term reduction in the prevalence of eating disorders and disordered eating behaviors (e.g., bulimic symptoms, emotional eating, binge eating behaviors, drive for thinness; Jebeile et al., 2019). A critical factor contributing to these findings is length of engagement with treatment, which highlights the importance of more nuanced understanding of patients who discontinue treatment.

Binge Eating Disorder

BED is characterized by distinct episodes in which an individual consumes objectively large quantities of food in a discrete period of time. This overeating is accompanied by a sense of loss of control and is not associated with recurrent use of compensatory behaviors such as self-induced vomiting, laxative or diuretic use, prolonged fasting, or overexercise (American Psychiatric Association, 2013). Although loss-of-control eating has been established as a consistent marker of binge-eating behavior, quantifying "large quantities of food" has proven more difficult, in particular among children and adolescents (Wilfley et al., 2016; Wolkoff et al., 2011).

Typical onset of BED occurs during adolescence (American Psychiatric Association, 2013), and an estimated 2% to 2.5% of adolescents meet criteria for the disorder (Field et al., 2012; Smink et al., 2014). These estimates do not account for the many more adolescents who engage in subclinical levels of binge eating behaviors (Lee-Winn et al., 2016; Tanofsky-Kraff, 2008).

One form of subclinical BED that merits additional clinical attention is *emotional overeating* (Masheb & Grilo, 2006). Emotional overeating involves eating large amounts of food as a means of coping with negative emotions such as attempting to soothe or suppress stress, fear, loneliness, or boredom. Emotional overeating often leads to a cycle in which eating large amounts of food in response to emotional triggers leads to additional distress over and beyond the initial negative emotion.

Despite not meeting diagnostic criteria for frequency or duration, subclinical BED and emotional overeating are associated with medical and psychological complications (Gianini et al., 2013; Sonneville et al., 2013; Trace et al., 2012). For example, loss-of-control eating is associated with increased risk for obesity and related comorbidities (e.g., hypertension, type 2 diabetes; J. E. Mitchell, 2016; Tanofsky-Kraff et al., 2009). Moreover, binge eating and emotional overeating behaviors are associated with increased risk for mood and anxiety disorders as well as decreased self-esteem, all of which are linked to pediatric obesity (Grilo et al., 2009; Kessler et al., 2013).

Given the disproportionate prevalence of pediatric obesity in communities of color, it is important to evaluate disordered eating patterns among racial/ethnic minority youth (Hammerle et al., 2016; Stice et al., 2017). BED has been identified as the most common specific eating disorder among non-Hispanic Black adolescents (J. Y. Taylor et al., 2007), and subclinical binge eating behaviors are more common among this group when compared with their non-Hispanic White counterparts (Marques et al., 2011). Even though non-Hispanic Black adolescents report higher prevalence of binge eating symptoms, they express less distress associated with these behaviors (Lee-Winn et al., 2016). Thus, it is not surprising that these youth are less likely to seek treatment for their maladaptive eating patterns. As such, it is important that health care clinicians be attuned to cultural differences that may influence clinical presentations that do not align with traditional diagnostic criteria.

Atypical Anorexia

In recognition of the clinical distress that can exist in the absence of meeting full diagnostic criteria, the *DSM-5* (American Psychiatric Association, 2013) introduced a revised category, "other specified feeding and eating disorders" (OSFED). This category of subclinical presentations includes five specific examples of disordered feeding and eating behaviors. In addition to BED of low frequency and/or limited duration (as described earlier), OSFED also recognizes that restrictive eating disorders require clinicians and researchers to look beyond low weight as a primary indicator of malnourishment (Garber, 2018). Atypical anorexia nervosa (AAN) includes all clinical features of AN (i.e., restricting energy intake, intense fear of gaining weight, disturbance in one's experience of body weight or shape; American Psychiatric Association, 2013). The distinguishing factor is that despite significant weight loss, the individual's presenting weight is within or above the normal range for BMI. Individuals diagnosed with AAN may also include those whose bodies have resisted weight loss despite caloric deprivation. The risks of medical and psychiatric instability (in particular, body image distortion) are similar for AN and AAN (Freizinger et al., 2022; Sawyer et al., 2016).

Studies suggest that recent weight loss is a more accurate indicator of restrictive eating disorder than crossing a lower BMI threshold (E. K. Hughes et al., 2017). Expanding criteria to consider individuals in higher weight bodies will certainly lead to more patients meeting criteria for AAN (Harrop et al., 2021). In fact, estimates indicate that adolescents with a history of overweight or obesity represent almost 40% of patients seeking treatment for serious restrictive eating disorders (Lebow, Sim, et al., 2015).

Adolescents with overweight or obesity face specific challenges in the context of eating disorder assessment and treatment as well as overall experience (Freizinger et al., 2022). These youth may be applauded by friends, family, and health care professionals for significant weight loss. Furthermore, clinicians may view weight loss as a positive health outcome and fail to assess for disordered eating. Meanwhile, weight loss methods may include severe dietary restriction, periods of starvation, use of self-induced vomiting, use of diet pills, and/or laxatives, or compulsive and excessive exercise (Golden et al., 2016).

Even in light of other symptoms indicating a diagnosis of AAN, the distress these youth experience may not be viewed with the same urgency or concern compared with adolescents with lower weights. In fact, their symptoms often go unrecognized, untreated, or undertreated (Bohrer et al., 2017; Harrop et al., 2021; Kennedy et al., 2017). The consequences of this disparity are poorer medical and psychological outcomes (Sawyer et al., 2016).

Restrictive eating has long been considered a disorder of non-Hispanic White females; however, males may be particularly vulnerable to more atypical presentations given that premorbid obesity is a risk factor for the development of disordered eating in males (Limbers et al., 2018). Likewise, research suggests there are higher rates of AAN in adolescents who identify as gender diverse or gender nonconforming (Mitchison et al., 2020). To date, studies on AAN largely have failed to report race, ethnicity, and socioeconomic status (Harrop et al., 2021), underscoring a need to represent the experiences of all people in research. Mitchison and colleagues (2014) argued that eating disorders seem to be increasing most in populations previously thought to be least at risk. Therefore, future research and clinical interventions must be more inclusive of sexual, gender, socioeconomic, racial, and ethnic diversity.

TREATMENT APPROACHES FOR DISORDERED EATING BEHAVIORS

Evidence-based therapies have demonstrated varying levels of efficacy in reducing disordered eating behaviors among youth (Lock, 2015; Rosen & The Committee on Adolescence, 2010; Tanofsky-Kraff et al., 2014). These treatments include family-based treatment (FBT), cognitive behavior therapy (CBT), and dialectical behavior therapy (DBT).

Family-Based Treatment

FBT, also known as the *Maudsley approach*, is the first-line approach to adolescent eating disorders. This outpatient intervention is for adolescents who are medically stable, and it requires significant involvement of parental caregivers (Lock & Le Grange, 2015). A central tenet of FBT is that neither adolescent nor parent are to blame for the eating disorder.

In the beginning phase of FBT, parental caregivers are guided by the therapist (in a nonauthoritarian fashion) to take charge of nutritional rehabilitation and weight recovery; they make all eating-related decisions for the adolescent. Then, as appropriate, control over eating is gradually returned to the adolescent. The final phase of FBT is implemented once the adolescent no longer exhibits symptoms of disordered eating and focuses on helping the adolescent resume an age-appropriate level of autonomy while addressing other mental health concerns.

FBT has been used to treat BN and OSFED, but it has been used most effectively to treat AN. Because of the similarities in presentation between adolescents with AN and AAN, researchers have suggested that FBT may be a helpful treatment strategy for patients with AAN (E. K. Hughes et al., 2017; Moskowitz & Weiselberg, 2017). However, determining appropriate treatment outcomes (e.g., reaching a goal weight, weight recovery, weight maintenance, need for weight gain) for youth with overweight or obesity has proven challenging (Dimitropoulos et al., 2019). Additional research is needed to inform adaptations of FBT for AAN. Similarly, there is scant research on applying FBT to treat BED.

Cognitive Behavior Therapy

Parental involvement in eating disorder treatment is not always practical or appropriate. CBT has been proposed as an alternative treatment when FBT is not feasible (Vogel et al., 2021). Most data supporting the application of CBT to treat disordered eating come from studies of adults; CBT is considered a first-line approach for adults with BN and BED (Freizinger et al., 2022). More recently, CBT has been enhanced to address transdiagnostic eating disorders in adults as well as adolescents (Dalle Grave, Eckhardt, et al., 2019).

CBT–Enhanced (CBT-E) was developed to help individuals achieve a healthy weight by addressing the psychopathology that overlays all eating disorders (Fairburn et al., 2003). Instead of taking a universal approach, CBT-E is highly individualized and focuses on specific mechanisms hypothesized to maintain the disorder. CBT-E is also highly collaborative, and patients are encouraged to prioritize treatment and actively participate in the process of change (Dalle Grave, Eckhardt, et al., 2019). Modifications for youth include techniques that support motivation while respecting the patient's developing autonomy (Dalle Grave, Sartirana, & Calugi, 2019). To date, there is limited evidence that CBT-E is efficacious for youth diagnosed with BED or AAN (Hilbert et al., 2020; Moskowitz et al., 2014; Moskowitz & Weiselberg, 2017).

Dialectical Behavior Therapy

DBT (Linehan, 1993a, 1993b), which was originally developed as a treatment for adults diagnosed with borderline personality disorder, has shown significant promise as a modified treatment for disordered eating (Reilly et al., 2020; Safer & Jo, 2010; Safer et al., 2009). DBT incorporates cognitive behavioral techniques and mindfulness-based strategies to improve emotion regulation, interpersonal effectiveness, and distress tolerance (see Table 13.1 for a sampling of DBT skills).

Proponents of the application of DBT to treat eating disorders highlight the association with high levels of emotion dysregulation as well as the frequent co-occurrence of impulsive behaviors such as substance use, non-suicidal self-injury, and suicidal behaviors (Kamody et al., 2019; Lavender et al., 2015). Furthermore, DBT, by design, focuses on multiple problem areas through the introduction of skills that have wide-ranging applications as opposed to exclusive focus on disordered eating behaviors (Vogel et al., 2021). For example, Kamody and colleagues (2020) found that distress tolerance skills, such as self-soothing (see Table 13.2), were rated as most helpful to youth engaging in binge eating behaviors. Another interesting

TABLE 13.1. Sample of Dialectical Behavioral Therapy Skills

Acronym	Skill	Description of skill
PLEASE	Treat **P**hysical I**l**lness Balanced **E**ating Avoid Mood **A**ltering Drugs Balanced **S**leep Get **E**xercise	*Emotion regulation* skill that helps with reducing emotional vulnerability and reactivity to facilitate quicker recovery during stressful situations
DEAR MAN	**D**escribe **E**xpress **A**ssert **R**einforce **M**indful **A**ppear Confident **N**egotiate	*Interpersonal effectiveness* skill aimed to assist in effectively getting needs met in a healthy and productive manner
GIVE	Be **G**entle Act **I**nterested **V**alidate Use an **E**asy Manner	*Interpersonal effectiveness* skill used to help with communication that fosters maintenance of relationships
FAST	**F**air No **A**pologies **S**tick to Values **T**ruthful	*Interpersonal effectiveness* skill used to maintain self-respect and increase self-esteem
Wise Mind ACCEPTS	**A**ctivities **C**ontributing **C**omparisons **E**motions **P**ushing Away **T**houghts **S**ensations	*Distress tolerance* skill used to distract oneself from difficult situations or emotional pain when one cannot immediately change them

Note. This table was developed on the basis of information presented in Rathus and Miller (2014) and A. L. Miller et al. (2006).

line of research has examined the use of DBT skills as an adjunctive treatment to FBT to increase adaptive coping and self-regulation (Peterson et al., 2020; Reilly et al., 2020).

Medications

Research on the role of psychiatric medications in adolescents presenting with disordered eating is limited. There is minimal empirical evidence for use of medications in the treatment of AN, and evidence for pharmacological treatment of AAN is even more scarce. Selective serotonin reuptake inhibitors (SSRIs) are especially ineffective in the acute, malnourished state of AN, even for treatment of anxiety and depression (Moskowitz & Weiselberg, 2017). It stands to reason that efficacy profiles may be better in individuals experiencing AAN, because they are at a higher weight. However, because

TABLE 13.2. Distress Tolerance: Self-Soothe With the Six Senses

Use your six senses to soothe negative emotions and prevent a tough situation from becoming worse. Below are some examples for each sense. Feel free to add your own self-soothing strategies!

Sense	Examples	Symbol
Touch	• Take a hot bath or cold shower • Rub lotion onto your body • Wrap up in a soft blanket • Stand outside and feel the breeze • _____	
Taste	• Eat a favorite healthy food • Suck on a piece of hard candy • Chew a minty or fruity gum • Sip an herbal tea or flavored water • _____	
Sight	• Watch a sunrise or sunset • Take a hike and observe nature • Look through a picture book of your favorite vacation spot • Go people-watching • _____	
Smell	• Smell fresh flowers • Use your favorite perfume or cologne • Inhale the aroma from a cup of coffee • Light a scented candle • _____	
Hearing	• Listen to your favorite song • Listen to a sound machine • Hum or sing a soothing tune out loud • Pay attention to sounds in nature • _____	
Movement	• Go for a walk or run • Practice yoga or stretching • Rock yourself gently • Dance • _____	

Note. This table was developed on the basis of information presented in Rathus and Miller (2014).

of their relative state of malnourishment, use of SSRIs should be limited. Atypical antipsychotics, mainly olanzapine (Zyprexa), have been proposed to treat severe cases of adolescent AN (Boachie et al., 2003; Dennis et al., 2006), although effectiveness was not demonstrated in a metanalysis (Dold et al., 2015). Furthermore, experts caution against the use of atypical antipsychotics in patients with AAN because of the potential for significant weight gain and cardiometabolic side effects (Moskowitz & Weiselberg, 2017).

SSRIs and tricyclic antidepressants have been associated with declines in symptoms of BN and BED (Moskowitz & Weiselberg, 2017). Topiramate (e.g.,

Qudexy XR, Topamax) has also been shown to reduce binge eating behavior and weight in adults (McElroy et al., 2007), but a case series showed a risk for development or exacerbation of eating disorder symptoms after the initiation of the drug in a sample of adolescents (Lebow, Chuy, et al., 2015). Finally, lisdexamfetamine dimesylate (Vyvanse) has been approved to treat BEDs in adults. This central nervous system stimulant is thought to act by suppressing appetite, increasing dopamine, and reducing impulsivity and inattention that may contribute to loss of control eating (V. R. Johnson et al., 2020). Additional research is required to better understand the potential for medications to address the intersection of pediatric obesity and eating disorders.

BODY IMAGE AND WEIGHT PERCEPTION

A common thread across pediatric obesity and eating disorders is body image. Children and adolescents with obesity express greater concern about weight, and more dissatisfaction with their body image, compared with other youth with normal weight (Harriger & Thompson, 2012). Likewise, many youth with restrictive eating disorders express body image distortion and fear of gaining weight. It is interesting that, although body image disturbance is not a diagnostic criterion for BED, many clinicians and researchers argue that individuals with BED experience overvaluation of weight and shape, which may be associated with greater eating pathology (Grilo, 2013). In fact, studies have shown that an overemphasis on weight and body shape is associated with weight gain and poor perception of physical health (Kamody et al., 2018; Thurston et al., 2017).

Behavioral health specialists are in an ideal position to assess how body image affects healthy and unhealthy lifestyle behaviors (Cadieux et al., 2016). Screening and monitoring of body image concerns, weight misperception, and eating pathology are key aspects of clinical practice in a pediatric weight management setting (Decaluwé & Braet, 2004; Jebeile et al., 2021; S. A. Taylor et al., 2018). Neumark-Sztainer (2009) made the following five recommendations for health care professionals to help prevent obesity and eating disorders in youth:

1. Provide education on the counterproductive nature of unhealthy weight control behaviors and the importance of healthy eating and physical activity behaviors that can be maintained on a regular basis.

2. Discourage body dissatisfaction as a motivator for change; instead, encourage nurturing of the current body through healthy eating, physical activity, and positive self-talk.

3. Encourage regular and enjoyable family meals.

4. Discourage family engagement in weight talk; instead, encourage a focus on achieving a healthy body and mind through healthy eating, physical activity, and positive self-talk.

5. Acknowledge previous experiences of weight stigma and bias.

OUTCOME OF THE CLINICAL CASE

Because of his endorsement of binge eating behaviors and co-occurring internalizing presentation, Prentice was referred to participate in the Emotional Overeating Intervention, a 10-week DBT skills-based group (Pluhar et al., 2018). This intervention is developmentally and culturally tailored to treat adolescent binge eating behaviors in the context of associated health concerns while also providing generalizable therapeutic strategies (Kamody et al., 2019).

During his Emotional Overeating Intervention intake, Prentice expressed frustration and anger that he was not considered a candidate for osteotomy because of his excess weight. He also expressed sadness that even though bariatric surgery was a viable means to lose enough weight, the approval process would take several months. He said that this would be lost time during which he could be exercising to improve his health. Prentice shared that overeating had become a primary coping strategy for his negative emotions and that urges to binge were particularly strong immediately after medical appointments. He stated that his goals for participating in the Emotional Overeating Intervention were to gain more control of his eating and find other ways to manage his negative emotions.

Prentice participated in the group intervention with four similar-age peers. During weekly sessions, he disclosed how hard it was to accept his health conditions and how he spent a lot of time thinking about how unfair his life is. He also talked about his dissatisfaction with his body and said that every time he saw himself in a mirror, he wished for a smaller body. The Emotional Overeating Intervention therapist noted that Prentice was incredibly empathic with other group members, although he frequently made comments that no one had it as bad as he did.

Prentice was observed to have a particularly difficult time with the DBT distress tolerance skill of Radical Acceptance. This skill involves accepting one's reality as it is, with no judgment (A. L. Miller et al., 2006). He was not able to identify how his emotional distress, need for surgery on his leg,

(continues)

OUTCOME OF THE CLINICAL CASE *(Continued)*

and eating behaviors were all interconnected. He continued to focus on the unfairness of his situation and discontinued the group after the fifth session. Prentice did continue to attend appointments at the pediatric weight management clinic and was referred for individual therapy in the community to address his symptoms of depression. He ultimately was approved for bariatric surgery 9 months after his initial appointment.

CONCLUSION

Given their experiences of body dissatisfaction and encouragement from family, friends, health care practitioners, and society to lose weight, adolescents with obesity are particularly vulnerable to the development of disordered eating behaviors. However, this does not imply that every young person engaged in pediatric weight management will develop an eating disorder. Current evidence suggests that adolescents seeking treatment for obesity should be monitored for disordered eating patterns in a context of supervision and positive support from health care professionals.

KEY POINTS

- Psychologists and behavioral health specialists working with youth with obesity should be attuned to disordered eating patterns, even subclinical presentations.

- Ideal body image is influenced by many factors, in particular, culture. It is important that clinicians not make assumptions about individuals' satisfaction or dissatisfaction with their weight or body shape.

THINKING OUTSIDE THE BOX

What are the arguments for and against assessing every child and adolescent with obesity for binge eating disorder?

14

ADVERSE AND TRAUMATIC EXPERIENCES

CLINICAL CASE INTRODUCTION

Jane is a 10-year-old non-Hispanic White female who presented to an outpatient interdisciplinary pediatric obesity clinic with her grandfather for health and behavior intervention in response to her excess weight. Her body mass index at the initial psychological visit in the clinic was 42.23, which is over the 99th percentile for her age and sex and falls in the severe obesity, or Class 3, range. Her grandfather reports concerns regarding the limited number of foods Jane eats. Developmentally, she was born on time but had significant complications related to breathing issues and liver problems shortly after birth. She reportedly spent 3 weeks in the neonatal intensive care unit and 3 months in the newborn nursery. Her grandfather reports previous concerns regarding her development, such as limited verbalizations, but her biological parents refused early intervention services. Jane currently lives with her grandfather, aunt, uncle, and siblings. She was

(continues)

https://doi.org/10.1037/0000401-014
Psychological Approaches to the Treatment of Pediatric Obesity, by C. S. Lim and E. T. Burton

CLINICAL CASE INTRODUCTION (Continued)

recently removed from her biological parents' care because of suspected child abuse and neglect toward Jane and her siblings. Jane's grandfather reports current financial concerns, specifically, food insecurity. Her school and academic functioning is unclear, but it is suspected she has not been attending school or receiving intervention services.

With regard to eating, Jane's grandfather reports that Jane eats only rice and gravy or mashed potatoes and gravy for every meal. The family suspects that was the only food she was given, or that was available, when she was living with her parents. Her grandfather reports they have gradually been trying to present her with new foods and foods from a variety of food groups, despite their current food insecurity. Jane displays significantly delayed speech and language. Throughout the initial visit, she made one-syllable sounds. Jane also engages in developmentally delayed behavior–she was observed during one clinic session sitting and crawling on the floor, and she chewed on a clothes hanger. She does respond appropriately to simple verbal directions provided by her grandfather (e.g., "sit in chair"). Her grandfather expresses concerns regarding her self-care behaviors, such as toileting and hygiene. He denies a history of Jane engaging in self-injurious behaviors or expressing homicidal or suicidal ideation, intent, or plan. Jane has no history of outpatient or inpatient psychological or psychiatric services.

ADVERSE CHILDHOOD EXPERIENCES

Adverse childhood experiences (ACEs) are intense, stressful, and traumatic events that occur before a child reaches adulthood (U.S. Centers for Disease Control and Prevention, 2022a). Broadly put, ACEs can include a variety of experiences, but most commonly they are considered one or more of the following: recurrent maltreatment (physical, emotional and sexual abuse, and neglect), household dysfunction (witnessing violence between parents or caregivers, parental separation, incarceration or substance abuse of a household member, mental illness, and suicide attempt or completion by a family member), and witnessing or being exposed to community violence (Chu & Chu, 2021).

Research has found that ACEs predict an increased risk of obesity in adolescence and into adulthood (Chu & Chu, 2021). The type and number of ACEs experienced appear to be important; specifically, experiencing sexual or physical abuse and being exposed to multiple ACEs increases the risk of developing obesity in childhood (Schroeder et al., 2021). Theories that explain associations between ACEs and obesity risk implicate ACEs as affecting both psychosocial and neuroendocrine systems, which leads to impairment in self-regulation, appetite, psychological symptoms, and disruptions to the family system. Individual aspects of the adverse or traumatic experience may also be important to consider in the context of prevention and treatment of pediatric obesity. For example, harsh discipline and physical abuse may occur in the context of family meals or the child trying new foods, which could lead to avoidance of specific foods or a reexperiencing of trauma symptoms while receiving pediatric weight management treatment. Neglect specific to limited availability and/or variety of food would also be important to consider. For example, *food insecurity*, defined as lack of consistent access to adequate food because of limited financial and physical resources (Coleman-Jensen et al., 2021), is associated with higher weight status in infants and children (St. Pierre et al., 2022). Caregiver *medical neglect*, whereby children experience a lack of access to preventative and regular medical care, also may result in increased weight gain and exacerbation of developmental, physical, and mental health conditions. In summary, screening and assessing for ACEs in the prevention and treatment of pediatric obesity is important.

TEASING, BULLYING, AND WEIGHT STIGMA

As defined previously, recurrent emotional abuse is considered an ACE. Name calling, criticism, and humiliation are all harmful for child development, and children with overweight or obesity are at increased risk for experiencing teasing and bullying targeted at weight and/or body shape. Youth may experience emotional abuse in a variety of settings and contexts, including home, school, and the community (Puhl & Lessard, 2020). These experiences can result in stress and trauma symptoms that influence emotional, social, and psychological functioning, as well as affect motivation and engagement in health behaviors to prevent and treat pediatric obesity (Pont et al., 2017). Thus, experiencing bullying and weight stigma can be conceptualized as adverse or traumatic experiences for youth.

Bullying has been defined as repeated undesirable behaviors involving an imbalance of power toward the perpetrator or group of perpetrators and can take on various forms, including verbal (e.g., name calling), physical (e.g., hitting), and relational (e.g., social exclusion) behaviors (Koyanagi et al., 2020). In addition, bullying leads to negative emotions (e.g., sadness, depression, low self-esteem, and poor body image) and increases the risk of engaging in disordered eating behaviors, such as emotional eating and binge eating, as well as avoidance of engagement in physical activity (Puhl & Luedicke, 2012). Decades of research have revealed that experiencing bullying puts youth at risk for poor physical and psychological health outcomes (Koyanagi et al., 2020). *Weight stigma* has been recognized as comprising negative beliefs that are based on weight, and it often leads to actions against a person (Haqq et al., 2021). Weight stigma arises from negative personal attitudes and views about obesity and individuals with overweight or obesity (e.g., that they are lazy, have no willpower) and is recognized as being driven by a disregard for the complex etiology of obesity (Haqq et al., 2021). Children and adolescents with overweight or obesity experience weight stigma from multiple sources, including parents/caregivers, peers, teachers, media and entertainment outlets, and health care providers (Puhl & Heuer, 2010). In the community, they may also experience strangers making negative comments about their body shape, size, and weight. Some individuals have described weight stigma as the last socially accepted form of discrimination (Budd et al., 2011) because of the continued misperception that disparaging those who are overweight and obese, including children, will motivate them to lose weight. However, there is evidence that youth with overweight or obesity experience more weight stigma, which increases the risk of future weight gain (Ma et al., 2021); thus, associations between weight stigma and obesity risk appear to be bidirectional.

CHRONIC STRESS

Stress has also been recognized by The Obesity Society (2015) as a contributor to obesity that is important to consider in efforts to prevent and treat pediatric obesity. Stress disturbs the equilibrium between the brain and nervous systems, and experiencing chronic stress during development can affect one's later physical and mental health; thus, children are considered to be at increased vulnerability (Pervanidou & Chrousos, 2011). Families under chronic stress—for example, because of poverty—may have difficulties integrating healthy lifestyle changes, for a variety of reasons (e.g., housing instability, food insecurity). Chronic stress experienced via structural racism and discrimination is also important to recognize. Structural racism, recognized as comprising inequitable systems based on race and ethnicity that exist in societies (Egede et al., 2023; see also Table 2.1, this volume) affects families in numerous ways, including limiting housing availability and opportunities for home ownership as well as access to quality health care, health insurance, employment, and income, all of which have been linked to increased stress and poor health outcomes, including increased risk of weight gain and obesity development (Yearby, 2018).

Behavioral and biological mechanisms have both been used to explain associations between stress and obesity. Individuals who experience stress are more likely to engage in eating for emotional comfort, select unhealthier foods, get inadequate sleep, and engage in more impulsive behaviors (Pervanidou & Chrousos, 2011), all of which are associated with weight gain. Sources of both acute and chronic stress are important to identify and incorporate into the prevention and treatment of pediatric obesity.

OTHER TRAUMATIC EXPERIENCES

Children who experience other acute traumatic experiences, such as natural disasters (e.g., tornadoes, hurricanes, floods), accidents (e.g., motor vehicle collisions, fires), community violence (e.g., gun-related crimes, gang activity), and the death of a loved one may also experience stress and trauma symptoms, which could put them at increased risk of engaging in unhealthy weight control behaviors and eventually lead to the development of overweight and obesity.

Natural Disasters

It has been estimated that more than 250 million people worldwide are affected by natural disasters each year (Terasaka et al., 2015). The impact of experiencing a natural disaster on the functioning of children and families is variable. Key factors appear to be specific exposures related to the disaster (e.g., proximity), sociodemographic factors, experiencing multiple negative impacts (e.g., loss of family income, loss of stable housing), personality characteristics, and experiencing deaths of close family and friends (Fong & Iarocci, 2020). The time immediately following a natural disaster is when youth are most likely to experience symptoms of posttraumatic stress disorder. However, the prevalence and severity of these symptoms tends to decrease over time (Terasaka et al., 2015).

Community Violence

Youth in the United States and other parts of the world are exposed to community violence, such as fights, assaults, or shootings, which influences their academic performance as well as their physical and mental health (David-Ferdon et al., 2016). One study found that more than 37% of U.S. youth lived less than 1 mile (1.6 km) from at least one gun-related homicide that had occurred over the past year (Kravitz-Wirtz et al., 2022). In addition, youth with racial/ethnic minoritized identities and/or those who live in communities with high levels of poverty or neighborhood disadvantage are more likely to be exposed to gun-related deaths. Exposure to gun-related violence, such as witnessing gun-related crimes, hearing gunshots, knowing or being a victim of a gun-related crime, or hearing about gun-related deaths and injuries, can result in chronic stress and symptoms of posttraumatic stress disorder in youth. Living in crime-prone areas has been recognized by The Obesity Society (2015) as a potential contributor to obesity development and maintenance and as an important social determinant of health by other pediatric professional associations (Hampl et al., 2023b). Thus, exposure to community violence and other crimes is an important factor for psychologists and other mental health providers to consider in their assessment of pediatric obesity, as well as in the selection of prevention and treatment strategies to implement.

Death and Loss

Children and adolescents are likely to experience the death or loss of important people in their lives, such as family members or friends; the likelihood of experiencing death or loss increases as youth age and are exposed to more life events (Fitzgerald et al., 2021). Youth cope with death in a variety of normative ways that are unique to their temperament and cultural practices and that at times are different from the way their parents, caregivers, or siblings cope with grief. It is important for psychologists and other mental health providers to be aware of typical ways children and adolescents cope with grief and how this may change throughout the course of development and through life experiences.

Providing psychoeducation to families about developmentally appropriate grief responses is often important. Experiencing multiple deaths of loved ones and witnessing traumatic deaths may exacerbate typical grief reactions. During the COVID-19 pandemic, many children experienced the deaths of friends and family. However, quarantine restrictions often impeded typical sources of comfort and support, such as attending funerals, engaging in rituals or cultural practices, or just being with friends and loved ones (Fitzgerald et al., 2021). In pediatric obesity medical clinics, families often describe changes in child eating habits occurring after a specific event, such as the death of a close family member. In addition, some children may experience prolonged grief or bereavement that affects their functioning in a variety of ways, including eating behaviors and engagement in physical activity (Torbic, 2011). For psychologists working in pediatric obesity prevention and treatment settings, screening for adverse, traumatic, and chronic stress experiences is important, as is assessing for symptoms associated with trauma- and stressor-related disorders, such as posttraumatic stress disorder.

EVIDENCE-BASED PSYCHOLOGICAL TREATMENTS TO CONSIDER

In addition to screening and assessment, the integration of evidence-based psychological prevention and treatments is important to address trauma and related experiences in pediatric obesity. First, there has been a call to develop and implement strategies to prevent all children from experiencing ACEs through social programs implemented in a variety of social ecological settings. These include, for example, community-based programs that improve household financial security, legislation that limits corporal punishment, and mentoring programs that connect children with role models in their community (Chu & Chu, 2021). Family-centered substance abuse treatment and community, state, and national policies that reduce violence (e.g., gun control, domestic violence), should also be considered. At the family level, teaching caregivers positive parenting skills to improve the child–caregiver relationship and reduce caregiver stress and burden would be important. Psychologists and other mental health providers could expose families to these skills in community-based and medical settings, such as primary care and specialty care clinics. The Incredible Years is an example of an empirically supported group-based parenting skills program designed for caregivers of children at various ages and is considered cost-effective (Pidano & Allen, 2015).

To successfully combat weight bias and stigma, multiple intervention strategies implemented at various socioecological levels have been recommended (Brownell et al., 2005). First, training teachers, employers, and health care providers about weight bias and related advocacy issues that occur in the physical and interpersonal environment is important. For psychologists and mental health providers working in pediatric obesity prevention and treatment settings, this could include advocating for appropriate medical equipment, such as chairs without armrests, or physical activities that accommodate the spectrum of athletic ability and body sizes and shapes.

Behavioral health specialists are uniquely qualified to role-model professional behavior to colleagues, staff, and trainees that is non-stigmatizing toward children with obesity and their families (Pont et al., 2017). Language and word choices used when interacting with patients and families should be neutral and respectful. Although person-first language has been encouraged, research suggests that clinicians should ask youth about their preferences for language when discussing weight-related health (Puhl, Himmelstein, et al., 2017). In other communications, such as clinical documentation, scientific writing, professional presentations, clinical case discussions, and media reporting, person-first language is critical to mitigate stigma, bias, and discrimination (Fisch et al., 2022; Obesity Action Coalition, 2022).

Screening for experiences related to teasing and bullying is key to psychosocial assessment of youth with obesity. If the child is currently experiencing bullying, psychologists should provide psychoeducation to caregivers and youth about school-based resources that may be available (e.g., school and district policies about bullying, community advocacy groups that can help with school-related support) and help families feel more comfortable talking with teachers and other school personnel about their concerns regarding bullying. Coaching caregivers and children about ways to bring up concerns regarding bullying is one tool that could be integrated into individual treatment in pediatric obesity prevention and treatment settings.

For youth who experience teasing and bullying, individual treatment focused on adaptive coping skills is indicated. Given research that children and adolescents who are bullied by others tend to demonstrate social skills deficits (Fox & Boulton, 2005), social skills training may also be a valuable intervention. Social skills training typically targets social impairments by focusing on increasing children's knowledge regarding social behaviors and rules as well as providing opportunities for children to practice various social skills in a supportive environment (Mikami et al., 2014).

For children and adolescents with clinically significant trauma and grief symptoms, trauma-focused evidence-based treatments, such as trauma-focused cognitive behavior therapy (TF-CBT; Cohen & Mannarino, 2015) or Alternative for Families: A Cognitive Behavior Therapy (AF-CBT; Kolko et al., 2011), may be warranted. The development of TF-CBT was informed by cognitive behavioral, attachment, developmental, neurobiological, family, and humanistic theoretical models, and the treatment includes psychoeducation, skills focused on parenting, relaxation, emotion and affect regulation, cognitive processing, trauma processing, in vivo exposures related to the trauma, combined parent–child sessions, and safety skills training (Cohen et al., 2017). AF-CBT is focused primarily on caregivers and provides training on self-regulation skills to reduce caregiver engagement in harmful or dangerous behaviors directed toward the child; these skills are then applied to the family context to improve the child's behavioral and social functioning (Kolko et al., 2011).

In addition to implementing these treatments before, during, or after pediatric weight management treatment, trauma-focused evidence-based treatments can be modified to incorporate aspects of psychological treatment for weight management. In individual treatment, TF-CBT is tailored on the basis of past traumas and exposures. It is therefore possible to incorporate aspects of the child's eating and physical activity behaviors in the context of the traumatic experience. This may be clinically indicated if, for example, the child experienced trauma in the context of eating or engaging in physical activity. Similar to TF-CBT, AF-CBT aims to identify specific, individualized problems of focus that can be integrated into treatment and monitored for improvement (Kolko et al., 2011). Thus, it is possible for healthy lifestyle behaviors to be incorporated into these treatments, and the cognitive and behavioral skills could also be applied to concepts that are consistent with weight management.

OUTCOME OF THE CLINICAL CASE

At Jane's initial evaluation, it was clear there were significant concerns related to neglect, trauma, and development. On the same day as their evaluation, Jane and her family met with the clinic social worker to address their financial concerns and food insecurity. Jane was also referred for consultation with specialists in developmental and behavioral pediatrics as well as speech therapy to determine what medical and therapy services were warranted. Jane's grandfather was encouraged to meet with the school she would be attending to determine what special educational and therapy services she would be able to receive in that setting. Finally, the family was assigned a case manager to assist them in coordinating and navigating the multiple appointments these referrals and recommendations generated.

During the course of Jane's treatment, her aunt and grandfather were awarded full custody of her and her siblings. The speech evaluation revealed that her expressive speech was at the 1 year, 9-month-old level. At school, she was given an Individualized Education Plan that provided for speech therapy, occupational therapy, and physical therapy services in that setting. In addition, she was able to obtain speech therapy and physical therapy services in the community.

(continues)

OUTCOME OF THE CLINICAL CASE (*Continued*)

In follow-up appointments with the pediatric obesity clinic, the family was encouraged to gradually yet continually expose Jane to new foods and support her learning of self-care skills. Her aunt and grandfather worked together to introduce healthier foods, in particular, fruits and vegetables. It became clear that Jane's previously restricted diet was related to limited exposure to diverse foods. One strategy the family found helpful was incorporating vegetables into foods Jane would already eat (e.g., adding pureed vegetables to gravy). They also worked on establishing a consistent routine for Jane and her siblings at home, which included time playing outside and being more physically active.

During a follow-up clinic with the psychologist, the family reported concerns regarding Jane wanting to eat all the time when she saw food. They also were concerned that she was sneaking food when family members were not supervising her in the kitchen. Taking into account her experience of neglect, trauma, and developmental concerns, psychoeducation was provided to the family regarding food being a source of comfort and Jane experiencing difficulties related to impulse control around food. The care team discussed the importance of stimulus control and steps the family could take to limit Jane's access to food more generally. Her grandfather, aunt, uncle, and siblings were on board with these approaches, and every family member helped implement the lifestyle-focused changes. The family was also interested in helping Jane continue to learn self-care skills to gradually increase her independence at home.

While meeting with the psychologist during follow-up clinic visits, the family was taught strategies to break down self-care skills into smaller steps and identify ones in which Jane could engage independently and others for which she needed more support according to her current level of functioning. The family was encouraged to provide praise and reinforcement when Jane was able to complete tasks successfully with minimal assistance. The combination of appropriate medical and therapy services, along with the family's supportive and encouraging implementation of structure, routine, and exposure to healthy lifestyle behaviors, contributed to gradual improvement of Jane's weight status. She also made significant improvements in her speech, academic, and self-care skills.

CONCLUSION

In the context of pediatric obesity prevention and treatment efforts, the assessment of adverse experiences and chronic stress is important, as are recognizing and understanding the potential effect these previous experiences may have on child health behaviors, self-esteem and body image, and coping mechanisms. Pediatric weight management providers should consider implementing trauma-informed care in medical and psychological treatment settings. Evidence-based treatments addressing trauma symptoms and many of the available treatments can be modified to incorporate eating and physical activity behaviors and weight management techniques to address comorbidity concerns.

KEY POINTS

- Adverse experiences and chronic stress influence the development and intractability of pediatric obesity.

- Psychologists and other mental health providers should be equipped to provide evidence-based prevention and treatment strategies that reduce chronic stress and trauma and address pediatric obesity.

THINKING OUTSIDE THE BOX

What are possible benefits and consequences of developing and implementing prevention and intervention programs that seek to simultaneously address both adverse childhood experiences and pediatric obesity?

15

FUTURE CLINICAL, RESEARCH, AND ADVOCACY DIRECTIONS

Pediatric obesity is a complex chronic medical condition that affects physical, psychological, emotional, and social functioning across many domains. These deleterious health effects exert their consequential influence across the life span, which translates to billions of dollars in health care expenses each year. As the prevalence and severity of pediatric obesity continue to rise, the public health implications become more pronounced.

The etiology of pediatric obesity is multifactorial, an outcome attributable to interacting biological characteristics and environmental exposures. The impact of pediatric obesity could also be due to weight stigma and discrimination youth experience in multiple settings. Children with obesity are more likely to experience teasing and bullying and are at risk of developing internalizing and externalizing symptoms. The experience of weight stigma and related discrimination could also expose youth to traumatic experiences. Weight bias also influences how researchers interpret and discuss their findings and how clinicians practice and treat youth and their families; thus, increased education, awareness, and modification of these biases are important. As research in the prevention and treatment of obesity and pediatric obesity

https://doi.org/10.1037/0000401-015
Psychological Approaches to the Treatment of Pediatric Obesity, by C. S. Lim and E. T. Burton

continues to advance, additional etiologies and potential prevention and treatment avenues will be identified. Future clinical and research directions related to psychological research and practice focused on pediatric obesity prevention and treatment are reviewed in the sections that follow.

INDIVIDUALIZED TREATMENT APPROACHES

Because of its chronicity, complexity, and the multiple domains of functioning obesity can affect, it is important that psychologists and other mental health care providers working in pediatric obesity prevention and treatment settings individualize treatment approaches to youth and their families as well as to their context (e.g., community). A one-size-fits-all approach will not work. In fact, the Etiology-Based Personalized Intervention Strategy Targeting Childhood Obesity (EPISTCO) has been proposed as a framework to guide the prevention and treatment of pediatric obesity (Motevalli et al., 2021). EPISTCO is described as an approach that focuses on specific lifestyle intervention strategies (e.g., eating, physical activity, sleep, psychological symptoms) based on the individual's specific etiology of obesity and individual and environmental characteristics that support and hinder weight management efforts. Psychological treatments targeting obesity, as well as medical and other health-related treatments (e.g., medication, surgery), should also be individualized for pediatric patients and their families. Psychologists and other mental health care providers should ensure that strengths of youth, caregivers, families, and communities are incorporated into prevention and treatment efforts. Innovative approaches such as precision medicine and precision nutrition aim to tailor prevention and treatment efforts to an individual on the basis of their genetic, biological, and environmental characteristics (Y. Wu et al., 2020). Evidence-informed ways that obesity treatments can be individualized will be an important avenue for future behavior health–focused clinical research.

TECHNOLOGICAL APPROACHES

Future pediatric obesity prevention and treatment efforts should continue to investigate innovative ways to incorporate aspects of technology. Telehealth has clear applications to the assessment and treatment of pediatric health conditions and has the potential to increase the amount of care provided and the number of patients who can be evaluated and treated through this modality (Cushing, 2017). The use of telehealth in the United States and across the globe increased substantially in response to the COVID-19 pandemic, and telehealth is expected to continue to play a large role in health care delivery post-pandemic (Thomas et al., 2022). Telehealth has been recognized as useful for treating and managing pediatric obesity (Cueto & Sanders, 2020), and researchers have been developing and evaluating group-based behavioral family pediatric obesity treatments delivered via telehealth for more than 10 years (A. M. Davis et al., 2011, 2013).

Advances in electronic health (eHealth) and mobile health (mHealth) have increased; this has been driven by increased rates of smartphone ownership, use of personal computers, and widespread access to high-speed internet services. For example, 95% of U.S. teenagers (i.e., 13- to 17-year-olds) report they have a smartphone or regular access to a smartphone (M. Anderson & Jiang, 2018). The accessibility of app-based health promotion and obesity prevention and treatment programs on phones and tablets has increased exponentially. However, many available apps do not incorporate evidence-based recommendations or target specific lifestyle behaviors, and their efficacy typically has not been evaluated before they are made accessible to youth and their families (Puig et al., 2019; Schoffman et al., 2013); thus, their ability to effectively prevent and treat pediatric obesity are currently questionable. In addition, there are concerns that youth who interact with apps that are not consistent with evidence-based recommendations could result in disordered eating and decreased physical activity behaviors, as well as decreased self-esteem and increased psychological symptoms.

For advances to be made in the implementation of telehealth, eHealth, and mHealth focused on pediatric obesity prevention and treatment, it is vital that clinical researchers specifically develop and evaluate the usability, engagement, and efficacy of telehealth and eHealth/mHealth applications for children and teens and ensure that these applications incorporate evidence-based strategies. In addition, psychologists and other health care providers should be aware of evidence-based apps and electronic approaches that have research support for their efficacy and that can be discussed and potentially used by families in pediatric obesity treatment settings. Conversely, providers should also attempt to stay up-to-date regarding electronic information and materials that are not evidence-based in order to educate families regarding tools that may not be recommended to supplement their care.

DIVERSITY, EQUITY, AND INCLUSION

In the prevention and treatment of pediatric obesity, issues specific to diversity, equity, and inclusion are critical and will continue to be in the future. Systemic racism and discrimination experienced by marginalized groups, and the impact of these experiences on health, including obesity, have been garnering increased focus. There is a need for future research and childhood obesity prevention and treatment efforts to consider links between experiences of discrimination and racism and health behaviors and outcomes (Mackey et al., 2022).

Gender and gender identity are critical areas in which more work will need to be conducted. For example, there is evidence that the psychosocial and educational consequences of obesity are more harmful to girls compared with boys (Crosnoe, 2007). In addition, the weight status of individuals who identify as transgender has become an increasing focus: Research has found that almost 60% of adults who identify as transgender have overweight or obesity (Sackey et al., 2021) and, for some patients, excess weight may limit options with regard to receiving approval to undergo gender-affirming surgical procedures (Martinson et al., 2020), or be prescribed gender-affirming medications. Future research focusing on health behaviors, weight status, body image, and gender identity development in children and adolescents will be an interesting area and will help inform appropriate modifications to future pediatric obesity prevention and treatment efforts.

Increasing access to pediatric obesity prevention and treatment efforts by children and families living in underresourced communities (e.g., low socioeconomic status, rural areas) will continue to be prominent issues related to diversity, equity, and inclusion that psychologists and other health care providers should incorporate into future clinical work and research. Telehealth and virtual treatment options may be one way to increase access. However, potential limitations, such as limited availability of high-speed internet access in rural communities, need to be considered so that disparities are not further exacerbated. The intersectionality of multiple-minoritized identities youth and families may experience, such as low income and identification as a member of a racial/ethnic minority group, is also important to consider. The additional intersection of overweight or obesity and experiencing weight-related stigma, as well as racial discrimination and bias, needs to be incorporated into future clinical research focused on the prevention and treatment of pediatric obesity (Mackey et al., 2022).

ADVOCACY

Currently, and in the future, psychologists and health care providers working to prevent and treat pediatric obesity should be prepared to participate in advocacy efforts at multiple levels. The ecological framework (Bronfenbrenner, 1979, 1995) can help guide advocacy efforts given that advocacy is needed in various settings, including the individual child and family, community, and health care, as well as at the local, state, and federal policy and legislation levels. In addition, advocacy should focus on structural efforts to reduce weight stigma and weight-related discrimination in a variety of social settings (e.g., school, housing, occupational, medical). The efficacy of advocacy efforts and related outcomes would also be important avenues for future research.

Psychologists are often in positions of power or authority such that they can provide education in various educational and health care settings about obesity being a chronic medical condition and the impact of weight stigma on children and families. When working with individual youth in a treatment setting, advocating for them to receive educational accommodations through the Individuals with Disabilities Education Act of 1990 (IDEA; Pub. L. 101-476) via 504 plans, which list resources a child with a disability needs in order to learn without barriers, where obesity is considered an "Other Health Impairment," if appropriate, may help improve individual educational and academic functioning.

With regard to the health care setting, a critical area for continued advocacy is related to insurance reimbursement for obesity treatment, as well as reimbursement for obesity screening and prevention efforts. Interdisciplinary and evidence-based pediatric outpatient medical treatment for obesity is often not covered by insurance providers and, when the treatment is covered, health care providers face numerous challenges to get their services reimbursed. Federal programs and policies are currently in place, such as through Medicaid's Early and Periodic Screening, Diagnostic and Treatment benefit, which covers obesity-related services that are medically necessary (Centers for Medicare & Medicaid Services, 2023). In addition, some states have passed legislation specific to insurance reimbursement for evidence-based interdisciplinary pediatric obesity treatment (e.g., Missouri's Biopsychosocial Treatment of Obesity; MO HealthNet Division, Missouri Department of Social Services, 2021).

In addition, while there have been advances in the number of medications approved by regulatory agencies for youth obesity treatment, insurance coverage for these medications is limited, and without insurance coverage most of the medications are costly for families (e.g., more than $1,000/month). Families and health care providers also face numerous obstacles and challenges associated with weight loss surgery. Although rates of insurance approval for adolescent bariatric surgery are improving (Gray et al., 2023), the process for obtaining coverage can be onerous for patients and families. Furthermore, pre- and postsurgical expenses (e.g., protein shakes, multivitamins) are often not covered by insurance providers. Given the health and socioeconomic disparities children with obesity and their families face, the cost of medications and surgery without insurance reimbursement is not possible for most patients. These barriers, which result from weight stigma and obesity discrimination, significantly limit the number of patients who receive weight loss medications or bariatric surgery, thereby perpetuating and exacerbating the ill effects of health disparities. Advocacy related to obesity being recognized as a chronic medical condition that is worthy of insurance coverage for evidence-based prevention efforts, weight loss treatments, medications, and medical procedures is vital to improve the health and psychological functioning of youth and families.

From a policy and legislative perspective, it is also important for psychologists and health care providers to be leaders in informing local, state, and federal officials regarding policies and legislation that is based on research evidence and reduces weight stigma. Obesity-focused legislation often experiences roadblocks to being passed and implemented. For example, available reviews of legislation demonstrates that fewer than 20% of proposed bills focused on adult obesity prevention are enacted (Donaldson et al., 2015). In addition, a large-scale national pediatric obesity prevention policy has yet to be enacted in the United States, but efforts have been made in other countries and specific cities within the United States that can help inform future work in this area. Overall, the lack of policy enactment suggests a need for increased collaboration between pediatric obesity specialists, such as psychologists, and the politicians who draft, propose, and vote on policies.

CONCLUSION

Pediatric obesity is a significant public health concern that is multifaceted in its development and treatment. There are numerous psychological factors and social determinants of health that are important to consider regarding the prevention and treatment of pediatric obesity and that influence youth and family engagement in treatment. Psychologists and other mental health care providers working in pediatric obesity prevention and treatment settings need to be trained in areas specific to the biological, genetic, medical, developmental, physical, social, and emotional experiences of pediatric patients and their families. Focusing on trainings and experiences that highlight the individualization of approaches and the need for reduction of weight stigma; technological advances related to the assessment, prevention, and treatment of obesity; issues specific to diversity, equity, and inclusion; and advocacy roles at multiple levels are needed so that current and future psychologists and health care providers focused on prevention and treatment of childhood obesity can work effectively to reduce the burden of this complex chronic disease on patients and families as well as on national and global health care systems.

KEY POINTS

- Psychologists and behavioral health specialists play a crucial role in the development and implementation of evidence-based pediatric obesity prevention and treatment strategies.

- Prevention and treatment strategies should be individualized and take into account psychological factors; social determinants of health; and issues related to weight bias, diversity, equity, and inclusion.

THINKING OUTSIDE THE BOX

What advocacy efforts can psychologists and behavioral health specialists engage in to improve prevention and treatment for pediatric obesity?

Appendix

The following resources may be helpful for psychologists and mental health clinicians who are working in various settings to prevent and treat pediatric obesity.

Association for Behavioral and Cognitive Therapies
https://www.abct.org
Society of Pediatric Psychology, Division 54 of the American Psychological Association
https://www.pedpsych.org
Society of Clinical Child and Adolescent Psychology, Division 53 of the American Psychological Association
https://sccap53.org/
The Obesity Action Coalition
https://www.obesityaction.org/
The Obesity Society
https://www.obesity.org
"Weight Bias in Clinical Care: Improving Health Care for Patients With Overweight and Obesity," a course by Rebecca M. Puhl and Young Suh, University of Connecticut Rudd Center for Food Policy & Obesity
https://uconnruddcenter.org/wp-content/uploads/sites/2909/2020/07/CME-Complete-with-links.pdf

References

Achenbach, T. M., & Edelbrock, C. (1991). *Child Behavior Checklist*. ASEBA.

Achenbach, T. M., Ivanova, M. Y., Rescorla, L. A., Turner, L. V., & Althoff, R. R. (2016). Internalizing/externalizing problems: Review and recommendations for clinical and research applications. *Journal of the American Academy of Child & Adolescent Psychiatry, 55*(8), 647–656. https://doi.org/10.1016/j.jaac.2016.05.012

Achenbach, T. M., & Rescorla, L. A. (2001). *Manual for the ASEBA School-Age Forms & Profiles*. University of Vermont, Research Center for Children, Youth, & Families.

Adams, T. D., Gress, R. E., Smith, S. C., Halverson, R. C., Simper, S. C., Rosamond, W. D., Lamonte, M. J., Stroup, A. M., & Hunt, S. C. (2007). Long-term mortality after gastric bypass surgery. *The New England Journal of Medicine, 357*(8), 753–761. https://doi.org/10.1056/NEJMoa066603

Agency for Healthcare Research and Quality. (2017). *National Healthcare Quality and Disparities Report: Chartbook on rural health care* (Publication No. 17[18]-0001-2-EF). https://www.ahrq.gov/sites/default/files/wysiwyg/research/findings/nhqrdr/chartbooks/qdr-ruralhealthchartbook-update.pdf

Alberga, A. S., Edache, I. Y., Forhan, M., & Russell-Mayhew, S. (2019). Weight bias and health care utilization: A scoping review. *Primary Health Care Research & Development, 20*, E116. https://doi.org/10.1017/S1463423619000227

Alqahtani, A., Elahmedi, M., Alqahtani, Y. A., & Al-Darwish, A. (2019). Endoscopic sleeve gastroplasty in 109 consecutive children and adolescents with obesity: Two-year outcomes of a new modality. *The American Journal of Gastroenterology, 114*(12), 1857–1862. https://doi.org/10.14309/ajg.0000000000000440

Alvarez, R., Bonham, A. J., Buda, C. M., Carlin, A. M., Ghaferi, A. A., & Varban, O. A. (2019). Factors associated with long wait times for bariatric surgery. *Annals of Surgery, 270*(6), 1103–1109. https://doi.org/10.1097/SLA.0000000000002826

Alvarez, R., Matusko, N., Stricklen, A. L., Ross, R., Buda, C. M., & Varban, O. A. (2018). Factors associated with bariatric surgery utilization among eligible candidates: Who drops out? *Surgery for Obesity and Related Diseases, 14*(12), 1903–1910. https://doi.org/10.1016/j.soard.2018.08.014

Alves, J. M., Yunker, A. G., DeFendis, A., Xiang, A. H., & Page, K. A. (2021). BMI status and associations between affect, physical activity and anxiety among U.S. children during COVID-19. *Pediatric Obesity, 16*(9), e12786. https://doi.org/10.1111/ijpo.12786

American Psychiatric Association. (2013). *Diagnostic and statistical manual of mental disorders* (5th ed.). https://doi.org/10.1176/appi.books.9780890425596

American Psychiatric Association. (2022). *Diagnostic and statistical manual of mental disorders* (5th ed., text rev.). https://doi.org/10.1176/appi.books.9780890425787

American Psychological Association. (2011). *Problem-Solving Skills Training (PSST)*. https://www.apa.org/pi/about/publications/caregivers/practice-settings/intervention/problem-skills

American Psychological Association. (2013). *Getting your weight under control*. https://www.apa.org/topics/obesity/weight-control

American Psychological Association. (2017). *What is cognitive behavioral therapy?* https://www.apa.org/ptsd-guideline/patients-and-families/cognitive-behavioral

American Psychological Association. (2018). *Clinical practice guideline for multicomponent behavioral treatment of obesity and overweight in children and adolescents: Current state of the evidence and research needs*. https://www.apa.org/obesity-guideline/clinical-practice-guideline.pdf

Aminian, A., Brethauer, S. A., Kirwan, J. P., Kashyap, S. R., Burguera, B., & Schauer, P. R. (2015). How safe is metabolic/diabetes surgery? *Diabetes, Obesity and Metabolism, 17*(2), 198–201. https://doi.org/10.1111/dom.12405

Aminian, A., & Nissen, S. E. (2020). Success (but unfinished) story of metabolic surgery. *Diabetes Care, 43*(6), 1175–1177. https://doi.org/10.2337/dci20-0006

Andela, S., Burrows, T. L., Baur, L. A., Coyle, D. H., Collins, C. E., & Gow, M. L. (2019). Efficacy of very low-energy diet programs for weight loss: A systematic review with meta-analysis of intervention studies in children and adolescents with obesity. *Obesity Reviews, 20*(6), 871–882. https://doi.org/10.1111/obr.12830

Anderson, L. M., Wong, N., Lanciers, S., & Lim, C. S. (2020). The relative importance of social anxiety facets on disordered eating in pediatric obesity. *Eating and Weight Disorders, 25*(1), 117–126. https://doi.org/10.1007/s40519-018-0526-x

Anderson, M., & Jiang, J.-J. (2018). *Teens, social media and technology*. Pew Research Center. https://www.pewresearch.org/internet/2018/05/31/teens-social-media-technology-2018/

Anderson, S. E., Cohen, P., Naumova, E. N., & Must, A. (2006). Association of depression and anxiety disorders with weight change in a prospective community-based study of children followed up into adulthood. *Archives of Pediatrics & Adolescent Medicine, 160*(3), 285–291. https://doi.org/10.1001/archpedi.160.3.285

Anderson, V., Anderson, P. J., Jacobs, R., & Smith, M. S. (2008). Development and assessment of executive function: From preschool to adolescence. In V. Anderson, R. Jacobs, & P. J. Anderson (Eds.), *Executive functions and the frontal lobes: A lifespan perspective* (pp. 123–154). Taylor & Francis.

Armstrong, S. C., Bolling, C. F., Michalsky, M. P., Reichard, K. W., Section on Obesity, Section on Surgery, Haemer, M. A., Muth, N. D., Rausch, J. C., Rogers, V. W., Heiss, K. F., Besner, G. E., Downard, C. D., Fallat, M. E., & Gow, K. W. (2019). Pediatric metabolic and bariatric surgery: Evidence, barriers, and best practices. *Pediatrics, 144*(6), e20193223. https://doi.org/10.1542/peds.2019-3223

Arterburn, D. E., Telem, D. A., Kushner, R. F., & Courcoulas, A. P. (2020). Benefits and risks of bariatric surgery in adults: A review. *JAMA, 324*(9), 879–887. https://doi.org/10.1001/jama.2020.12567

Ashiabi, G. S., & O'Neal, K. K. (2015). Child social development in context: An examination of some propositions in Bronfenbrenner's bioecological theory. *SAGE Open, 5*(2). https://doi.org/10.1177/2158244015590840

Assari, S. (2018). Family income reduces risk of obesity for White but not Black children. *Children, 5*(6), 73. https://doi.org/10.3390/children5060073

Aubert, S., Brazo-Sayavera, J., González, S. A., Janssen, I., Manyanga, T., Oyeyemi, A. L., Picard, P., Sherar, L. B., Turner, E., & Tremblay, M. S. (2021). Global prevalence of physical activity for children and adolescents; inconsistencies, research gaps, and recommendations: A narrative review. *International Journal of Behavioral Nutrition and Physical Activity, 18*(1), 81. https://doi.org/10.1186/s12966-021-01155-2

Baidal, J. A. W., Locks, L. M., Cheng, E. R., Blake-Lamb, T. L., Perkins, M. E., & Taveras, E. M. (2016). Risk factors for childhood obesity in the first 1,000 days: A systematic review. *American Journal of Preventive Medicine, 50*(6), 761–779. https://doi.org/10.1016/j.amepre.2015.11.012

Bailey, Z. D., Krieger, N., Agénor, M., Graves, J., Linos, N., & Bassett, M. T. (2017). Structural racism and health inequities in the USA: Evidence and interventions. *The Lancet, 389*(10077), 1453–1463. https://doi.org/10.1016/S0140-6736(17)30569-X

Ball, G. D. C., Ambler, K. A., Keaschuk, R. A., Rosychuk, R. J., Holt, N. L., Spence, J. C., Jetha, M. M., Sharma, A. M., & Newton, A. S. (2012). Parents as agents of change (PAC) in pediatric weight management: The protocol for the PAC randomized clinical trial. *BMC Pediatrics, 12*, 114. https://doi.org/10.1186/1471-2431-12-114

Barkley, R. A. (2013). *Defiant children: A clinician's manual for assessment and parent training* (3rd ed.). Guilford Press.

Barlow, S. E., & the Expert Committee. (2007). Expert Committee recommendations regarding the prevention, assessment, and treatment of child and adolescent overweight and obesity: Summary report. *Pediatrics, 120*(Suppl. 4), S164–S192. https://doi.org/10.1542/peds.2007-2329C

Barton, M., & the U.S. Preventive Services Task Force. (2010). Screening for obesity in children and adolescents: U.S. Preventive Services Task Force recommendation statement. *Pediatrics, 125*(2), 361–367. https://doi.org/10.1542/peds.2009-2037

Beck, A. R. (2016). Psychosocial aspects of obesity. *NASN School Nurse, 31*(1), 23–27. https://doi.org/10.1177/1942602X15619756

Bejarano, C. M., Marker, A. M., & Cushing, C. C. (2019). Cognitive–behavioral therapy for pediatric obesity. In R. D. Friedberg & J. K. Paternostro (Eds.), *Handbook of cognitive behavioral therapy for pediatric medical conditions* (pp. 369–383). Springer Nature. https://doi.org/10.1007/978-3-030-21683-2_23

Berge, J. M., Hanson-Bradley, C., Tate, A., & Neumark-Sztainer, D. (2016). Do parents or siblings engage in more negative weight-based talk with children and what does it sound like? A mixed-methods study. *Body Image, 18,* 27–33. https://doi.org/10.1016/j.bodyim.2016.04.008

Berge, J. M., Trofholz, A., Fong, S., Blue, L., & Neumark-Sztainer, D. (2015). A qualitative analysis of parents' perceptions of weight talk and weight teasing in the home environments of diverse low-income children. *Body Image, 15,* 8–15. https://doi.org/10.1016/j.bodyim.2015.04.006

Berge, J. M., Wall, M., Hsueh, T. F., Fulkerson, J. A., Larson, N., & Neumark-Sztainer, D. (2015). The protective role of family meals for youth obesity: 10-year longitudinal associations. *The Journal of Pediatrics, 166*(2), 296–301. https://doi.org/10.1016/j.jpeds.2014.08.030

Białek-Dratwa, A., Szczepańska, E., Szymańska, D., Grajek, M., Krupa-Kotara, K., & Kowalski, O. (2022). Neophobia—A natural developmental stage or feeding difficulties for children? *Nutrients, 14*(7), 1521. https://doi.org/10.3390/nu14071521

Białek-Dratwa, A., Szymańska, D., Grajek, M., Krupa-Kotara, K., Szczepańska, E., & Kowalski, O. (2022). ARFID—Strategies for dietary management in children. *Nutrients, 14*(9), 1739. https://doi.org/10.3390/nu14091739

Binks, M. (2016). The role of the food industry in obesity prevention. *Current Obesity Reports, 5*(2), 201–207. https://doi.org/10.1007/s13679-016-0212-0

Birch, L., Savage, J. S., & Ventura, A. (2007). Influences on the development of children's eating behaviours: From infancy to adolescence. *Canadian Journal of Dietetic Practice and Research, 68*(1), s1–s56.

Bishop, S. R., Lau, M., Shapiro, S., Carlson, L., Anderson, N. D., Carmody, J., Segal, Z. V., Abbey, S., Speca, M., Velting, D., & Devins, G. (2004). Mindfulness: A proposed operational definition. *Clinical Psychology: Science and Practice, 11*(3), 230–241. https://doi.org/10.1093/clipsy.bph077

Blake-Lamb, T., Boudreau, A. A., Matathia, S., Tiburcio, E., Perkins, M. E., Roche, B., Kotelchuck, M., Shtasel, D., Price, S. N., & Taveras, E. M. (2018). Strengthening integration of clinical and public health systems to prevent maternal–child obesity in the first 1,000 days: A collective impact approach. *Contemporary Clinical Trials, 65*, 46–52. https://doi.org/10.1016/j.cct.2017.12.001

Blanchet, R., Kengneson, C.-C., Bodnaruc, A. M., Gunter, A., & Giroux, I. (2019). Factors influencing parents' and children's misperception of children's weight status: A systematic review of current research. *Current Obesity Reports, 8*(4), 373–412. https://doi.org/10.1007/s13679-019-00361-1

Bleich, S. N., Segal, J., Wu, Y., Wilson, R., & Wang, Y. (2013). Systematic review of community-based childhood obesity prevention studies. *Pediatrics, 132*(1), e201–e210. https://doi.org/10.1542/peds.2013-0886

Boachie, A., Goldfield, G. S., & Spettigue, W. (2003). Olanzapine use as an adjunctive treatment for hospitalized children with anorexia nervosa: Case reports. *International Journal of Eating Disorders, 33*(1), 98–103. https://doi.org/10.1002/eat.10115

Bohrer, B. K., Carroll, I. A., Forbush, K. T., & Chen, P. Y. (2017). Treatment seeking for eating disorders: Results from a nationally representative study. *International Journal of Eating Disorders, 50*(12), 1341–1349. https://doi.org/10.1002/eat.22785

Boisvert, J. A., & Harrell, W. A. (2015). Integrative treatment of pediatric obesity: Psychological and spiritual considerations. *Integrative Medicine, 14*(1), 40–47. https://www.ncbi.nlm.nih.gov/pubmed/26770130

Bolling, C. F., Armstrong, S. C., Reichard, K. W., Michalsky, M. P., Section on Obesity, Section on Surgery, Haemer, M. A., Muth, N. D., Rausch, J. C., Rogers, V. W., Heiss, K. F., Besner, G. E., Downard, C. D., Fallat, M. E., & Gow, K. W. (2019). Metabolic and bariatric surgery for pediatric patients with severe obesity. *Pediatrics, 144*(6), e20193224. https://doi.org/10.1542/peds.2019-3224

Bonham, M. P., Dordevic, A. L., Ware, R. S., Brennan, L., & Truby, H. (2017). Evaluation of a commercially delivered weight management program for adolescents. *The Journal of Pediatrics, 185*, P73–P80.e3. https://doi.org/10.1016/j.jpeds.2017.01.042

Bornstein, S. R., Schuppenies, A., Wong, M. L., & Licinio, J. (2006). Approaching the shared biology of obesity and depression: The stress axis as the locus of gene–environment interactions. *Molecular Psychiatry, 11*(10), 892–902. https://doi.org/10.1038/sj.mp.4001873

Borzutzky, C., King, E., Fox, C. K., Stratbucker, W., Tucker, J., Yee, J. K., Kumar, S., Cuda, S., Sweeney, B., Kirk, S., & the POWER Work Group. (2021). Trends in prescribing anti-obesity pharmacotherapy for paediatric weight management: Data from the POWER Work Group. *Pediatric Obesity, 16*(1), e12701. https://doi.org/10.1111/ijpo.12701

Bouchard, M. E., Tian, Y., Linton, S., De Boer, C., O'Connor, A., Ghomrawi, H., & Abdullah, F. (2022). Utilization trends and disparities in adolescent bariatric surgery in the United States 2009–2017. *Childhood Obesity, 18*(3), 188–196. https://doi.org/10.1089/chi.2021.0201

Bourne, L., Mandy, W., & Bryant-Waugh, R. (2022). Avoidant/restrictive food intake disorder and severe food selectivity in children and young people with autism: A scoping review. *Developmental Medicine & Child Neurology, 64*(6), 691–700. https://doi.org/10.1111/dmcn.15139

Bowleg, L. (2012). The problem with the phrase *women and minorities*: Intersectionality—An important theoretical framework for public health. *American Journal of Public Health, 102*(7), 1267–1273. https://doi.org/10.2105/AJPH.2012.300750

Bozinovic, K., McLamb, F., O'Connell, K., Olander, N., Feng, Z., Haagensen, S., & Bozinovic, G. (2021). U.S. national, regional, and state-specific socioeconomic factors correlate with child and adolescent ADHD diagnoses pre-COVID-19 pandemic. *Scientific Reports, 11*(1), 22008. https://doi.org/10.1038/s41598-021-01233-2

Bozzola, E., Spina, G., Agostiniani, R., Barni, S., Russo, R., Scarpato, E., Di Mauro, A., Di Stefano, A. V., Caruso, C., Corsello, G., & Staiano, A. (2022). The use of social media in children and adolescents: Scoping review on the potential risks. *International Journal of Environmental Research and Public Health, 19*(16), 9960. https://doi.org/10.3390/ijerph19169960

Braveman, P. A., Arkin, E., Proctor, D., Kauh, T., & Holm, N. (2022). Systemic and structural racism: Definitions, examples, health damages, and approaches to dismantling. *Health Affairs, 41*(2), 171–178. https://doi.org/10.1377/hlthaff.2021.01394

Bronfenbrenner, U. (1979). *The ecology of human development: Experiments in nature and design*. Harvard University Press.

Bronfenbrenner, U. (1995). Developmental ecology through space and time: A future perspective. In P. Moen, G. H. Elder, Jr., & K. Lüscher (Eds.), *Examining lives in context: Perspectives on the ecology of human development* (pp. 619–647). American Psychological Association. https://doi.org/10.1037/10176-018

Broskey, N. T., Wang, P., Li, N., Leng, J., Li, W., Wang, L., Gilmore, L. A., Hu, G., & Redman, L. M. (2017). Early pregnancy weight gain exerts the strongest effect on birth weight, posing a critical time to prevent childhood obesity. *Obesity, 25*(9), 1569–1576. https://doi.org/10.1002/oby.21878

Brown, C. L., & Perrin, E. M. (2018). Obesity prevention and treatment in primary care. *Academic Pediatrics, 18*(7), 736–745. https://doi.org/10.1016/j.acap.2018.05.004

Brown, H. E., Pearson, N., Braithwaite, R. E., Brown, W. J., & Biddle, S. J. (2013). Physical activity interventions and depression in children and adolescents: A systematic review and meta-analysis. *Sports Medicine, 43*(3), 195–206. https://doi.org/10.1007/s40279-012-0015-8

Brown, L., Dolisca, S.-B., & Cheng, J. K. (2015). Barriers and facilitators of pediatric weight management among diverse families. *Clinical Pediatrics, 54*(7), 643–651. https://doi.org/10.1177/0009922814555977

Browne, N. T., Hodges, E. A., Small, L., Snethen, J. A., Frenn, M., Irving, S. Y., Gance-Cleveland, B., & Greenberg, C. S. (2022). Childhood obesity within the lens of racism. *Pediatric Obesity, 17*(5), e12878. https://doi.org/10.1111/ijpo.12878

Brownell, K. D., Puhl, R. M., Schwartz, M. B., & Rudd, L. (2005). *Weight bias: Nature, consequences, and remedies.* Guilford Press.

Buchanan, L., Rooks-Peck, C. R., Finnie, R. K. C., Wethington, H. R., Jacob, V., Fulton, J. E., Johnson, D. B., Kahwati, L. C., Pratt, C. A., Ramirez, G., Mercer, S. L., Glanz, K., & the Community Preventive Services Task Force. (2016). Reducing recreational sedentary screen time: A community guide systematic review. *American Journal of Preventive Medicine, 50*(3), 402–415. https://doi.org/10.1016/j.amepre.2015.09.030

Budd, G. M., Mariotti, M., Graff, D., & Falkenstein, K. (2011). Health care professionals' attitudes about obesity: An integrative review. *Applied Nursing Research, 24*(3), 127–137. https://doi.org/10.1016/j.apnr.2009.05.001

Bullock, A., Sheff, K., Moore, K., & Manson, S. (2017). Obesity and overweight in American Indian and Alaska Native children, 2006–2015. *American Journal of Public Health, 107*(9), 1502–1507. https://doi.org/10.2105/AJPH.2017.303904

Burki, T. (2022). Social media and misinformation in diabetes and obesity. *The Lancet: Diabetes & Endocrinology, 10*(12), P845. https://doi.org/10.1016/S2213-8587(22)00318-7

Burton, E. T., Jones, T. L., Smith, W. A., & Han, J. C. (2020). Psychosocial functioning after one year of interdisciplinary pediatric weight management. *Behavioral Medicine, 46*(2), 92–99. https://doi.org/10.1080/08964289.2019.1570073

Burton, E. T., Mackey, E. R., Reynolds, K., Cadieux, A., Gaffka, B. J., & Shaffer, L. A. (2020). Psychopathology and adolescent bariatric surgery: A topical review to support psychologists in assessment and treatment considerations. *Journal of Clinical Psychology in Medical Settings, 27*(2), 235–246. https://doi.org/10.1007/s10880-020-09717-5

Burton, E. T., & Smith, W. A. (2020). Mindful eating and active living: Development and implementation of a multidisciplinary pediatric weight management intervention. *Nutrients, 12*(5), 1425. https://doi.org/10.3390/nu12051425

Buscot, M.-J., Thomson, R. J., Juonala, M., Sabin, M. A., Burgner, D. P., Lehtimäki, T., Hutri-Kähönen, N., Viikari, J. S. A., Jokinen, E., Tossavainen, P., Laitinen, T., Raitakari, O. T., & Magnussen, C. G. (2018). BMI trajectories associated with resolution of elevated youth BMI and incident adult obesity. *Pediatrics, 141*(1), e20172003. https://doi.org/10.1542/peds.2017-2003

Cadieux, A., Getzoff Testa, E., Baughcum, A., Shaffer, L. A., Santos, M., Sallinen Gaffka, B. J., Gray, J., Burton, E. T., & Ward, W. L. (2016). Recommendations for psychologists in Stage III pediatric obesity program. *Children's Health Care, 45*(1), 126–145. https://doi.org/10.1080/02739615.2014.979919

Calcaterra, V., Cena, H., Pelizzo, G., Porri, D., Regalbuto, C., Vinci, F., Destro, F., Vestri, E., Verduci, E., Bosetti, A., Zuccotti, G., & Stanford, F. C. (2021). Bariatric surgery in adolescents: To do or not to do? *Children, 8*(6), 453. https://doi.org/10.3390/children8060453

Calpbinici, P., & Tas Arslan, F. (2019). Virtual behaviors affecting adolescent mental health: The usage of internet and mobile phone and cyberbullying. *Journal of Child and Adolescent Psychiatric Nursing, 32*(3), 139–148. https://doi.org/10.1111/jcap.12244

Carbone, L., Zebrack, B., Plegue, M., Joshi, S., & Shellhaas, R. (2013). Treatment adherence among adolescents with epilepsy: What really matters? *Epilepsy & Behavior, 27*(1), 59–63. https://doi.org/10.1016/j.yebeh.2012.11.047

Cardel, M. I., & Taveras, E. M. (2020). Let's not just dismiss the WW Kurbo app. *Childhood Obesity, 16*(1), 1–2. https://doi.org/10.1089/chi.2019.0222

Carr, A. (2019). Family therapy and systemic interventions for child-focused problems: The current evidence base. *Journal of Family Therapy, 41*(2), 153–213. https://doi.org/10.1111/1467-6427.12226

Chandrakumar, H., Khatun, N., Gupta, T., Graham-Hill, S., Zhyvotovska, A., & McFarlane, S. I. (2023). The effects of bariatric surgery on cardiovascular outcomes and cardiovascular mortality: A systematic review and meta-analysis. *Cureus, 15*(2), e34723. https://doi.org/10.7759/cureus.34723

Chew, C. S. E., Davis, C., Lim, J. K. E., Lim, C. M. M., Tan, Y. Z. H., Oh, J. Y., Rajasegaran, K., Chia, Y. H. M., & Finkelstein, E. A. (2021). Use of a mobile lifestyle intervention app as an early intervention for adolescents with obesity: Single-cohort study. *Journal of Medical Internet Research, 23*(9), e20520. https://doi.org/10.2196/20520

Childerhose, J. E., & Tarini, B. A. (2015). Understanding outcomes in adolescent bariatric surgery. *Pediatrics, 136*(2), e312–e314. https://doi.org/10.1542/peds.2015-0867

Chu, W. W.-e., & Chu, N.-F. (2021). Adverse childhood experiences and development of obesity and diabetes in adulthood—A mini review. *Obesity Research & Clinical Practice, 15*(2), 101–105. https://doi.org/10.1016/j.orcp.2020.12.010

Chubb, B., Gupta, P., Gupta, J., Nuhoho, S., Kallenbach, K., & Orme, M. (2021). Once-daily oral semaglutide versus injectable GLP-1 RAs in people with type 2 diabetes inadequately controlled on basal insulin: Systematic review and network meta-analysis. *Diabetes Therapy, 12*, 1325–1339. https://doi.org/10.1007/s13300-021-01034-w

Chung, M. S., Langouët, M., Chamberlain, S. J., & Carmichael, G. G. (2020). Prader–Willi syndrome: Reflections on seminal studies and future therapies. *Open Biology, 10*(9), 200195. https://doi.org/10.1098/rsob.200195

Clapp, B., Ponce, J., DeMaria, E., Ghanem, O., Hutter, M., Kothari, S., LaMasters, T., Kurian, M., & English, W. (2022). American Society for Metabolic and Bariatric Surgery 2020 estimate of metabolic and bariatric procedures performed in the United States. *Surgery for Obesity and Related Diseases, 18*(9), 1134–1140. https://doi.org/10.1016/j.soard.2022.06.284

Clément, K., van den Akker, E., Argente, J., Bahm, A., Chung, W. K., Connors, H., . . . & Yuan, G. (2020). Efficacy and safety of setmelanotide, an MC4R agonist, in individuals with severe obesity due to LEPR or POMC deficiency: Single-arm, open-label, multicentre, phase 3 trials. *The Lancet Diabetes & Endocrinology*, *8*(12), 960–970. https://doi.org/10.1016/S2213-8587(20)30364-8

Cobb, L. K., Appel, L. J., Franco, M., Jones-Smith, J. C., Nur, A., & Anderson, C. A. (2015). The relationship of the local food environment with obesity: A systematic review of methods, study quality, and results. *Obesity*, *23*(7), 1331–1344. https://doi.org/10.1002/oby.21118

Cohen, J. A., & Mannarino, A. P. (2015). Trauma-focused cognitive behavior therapy for traumatized children and families. *Child and Adolescent Psychiatric Clinics of North America*, *24*(3), 557–570. https://doi.org/10.1016/j.chc.2015.02.005

Cohen, J. A., Mannarino, A. P., & Deblinger, E. (2017). *Treating trauma and traumatic grief in children and adolescents* (2nd ed.). Guilford Press. https://doi.org/10.1080/07317107.2017.1375719

Coleman-Jensen, A., Rabbitt, M. P., Gregory, C. A., & Singh, A. (2021). *Household food security in the United States in 2020* (Economic Research Report No. 298). https://www.ers.usda.gov/webdocs/publications/102076/err-298.pdf

Cooksey-Stowers, K., Schwartz, M. B., & Brownell, K. D. (2017). Food swamps predict obesity rates better than food deserts in the United States. *International Journal of Environmental Research and Public Health*, *14*(11), 1366. https://doi.org/10.3390/ijerph14111366

Cooper, Z., Fairburn, C. G., & Hawker, D. M. (2003). *Cognitive–behavioral treatment of obesity*. Guilford Press.

Cortese, S., Angriman, M., Comencini, E., Vincenzi, B., & Maffeis, C. (2019). Association between inflammatory cytokines and ADHD symptoms in children and adolescents with obesity: A pilot study. *Psychiatry Research*, *278*, 7–11. https://doi.org/10.1016/j.psychres.2019.05.030

Cortese, S., & Castellanos, F. X. (2014). The relationship between ADHD and obesity: Implications for therapy. *Expert Review of Neurotherapeutics*, *14*(5), 473–479. https://doi.org/10.1586/14737175.2014.904748

Cortese, S., Moreira-Maia, C. R., St. Fleur, D., Morcillo-Peñalver, C., Rohde, L. A., & Faraone, S. V. (2016). Association Between ADHD and obesity: A systematic review and meta-analysis. *The American Journal of Psychiatry*, *173*(1), 34–43. https://doi.org/10.1176/appi.ajp.2015.15020266

Coto, J., & Graziano, P. A. (2022). Targeting pediatric obesity via a Healthy Lifestyle Summer Camp intervention: How necessary is a parenting component? *Childhood Obesity*, *18*(5), 350–359. https://doi.org/10.1089/chi.2021.0152

Cramer, P., & Steinwert, T. (1998). Thin is good, fat is bad: How early does it begin? *Journal of Applied Developmental Psychology*, *19*(3), 429–451. https://doi.org/10.1016/S0193-3973(99)80049-5

Craske, M. G. (2010). *Cognitive–behavioral therapy*. American Psychological Association.

Crocker, P. R., Bailey, D. A., Faulkner, R. A., Kowalski, K. C., & McGrath, R. (1997). Measuring general levels of physical activity: Preliminary evidence for the Physical Activity Questionnaire for Older Children. *Medicine & Science in Sports & Exercise, 29*(10), 1344–1349. https://doi.org/10.1097/00005768-199710000-00011

Crosnoe, R. (2007). Gender, obesity, and education. *Sociology of Education, 80*(3), 241–260. https://doi.org/10.1177/003804070708000303

Cuda, S., Censani, M., Joseph, M., Browne, N., & O'Hara, V. (2022). Pediatric obesity algorithm®: A clinical tool for treating childhood obesity. https://www.obesitymedicine.org/childhood-obesity

Cueto, V., & Sanders, L. M. (2020). Telehealth opportunities and challenges for managing pediatric obesity. *Pediatric Clinics of North America, 67*(4), 647–654. https://doi.org/10.1016/j.pcl.2020.04.007

Cueto, V., Wang, C. J., & Sanders, L. M. (2019). Impact of a mobile app–based health coaching and behavior change program on participant engagement and weight status of overweight and obese children: Retrospective cohort study. *JMIR mHealth and uHealth, 7*(11), e14458. https://doi.org/10.2196/14458

Cushing, C. C. (2017). eHealth applications in pediatric psychology. In M. C. Roberts & R. G. Steele (Eds.), *Handbook of pediatric psychology* (5th ed., pp. 201–211). Guilford Press.

Czepiel, K. S., Perez, N. P., Campoverde Reyes, K. J., Sabharwal, S., & Stanford, F. C. (2020). Pharmacotherapy for the treatment of overweight and obesity in children, adolescents, and young adults in a large health system in the US. *Frontiers in Endocrinology, 11*, 290. https://doi.org/10.3389/fendo.2020.00290

Dalen, J., Brody, J. L., Staples, J. K., & Sedillo, D. (2015). A conceptual framework for the expansion of behavioral interventions for youth obesity: A family-based mindful eating approach. *Childhood Obesity, 11*(5), 577–584. https://doi.org/10.1089/chi.2014.0150

Dalle Grave, R., Eckhardt, S., Calugi, S., & Le Grange, D. (2019). A conceptual comparison of family-based treatment and enhanced cognitive behavior therapy in the treatment of adolescents with eating disorders. *Journal of Eating Disorders, 7*(1), 42. https://doi.org/10.1186/s40337-019-0275-x

Dalle Grave, R., Sartirana, M., & Calugi, S. (2019). Enhanced cognitive behavioral therapy for adolescents with anorexia nervosa: Outcomes and predictors of change in a real-world setting. *International Journal of Eating Disorders, 52*(9), 1042–1046. https://doi.org/10.1002/eat.23122

Dalton, W. T. I., III, & Kitzmann, K. M. (2012). A preliminary investigation of stimulus control, self-monitoring, and reinforcement in lifestyle interventions for pediatric overweight. *American Journal of Lifestyle Medicine, 6*(1), 75–89. https://doi.org/10.1177/1559827611402582

Daniels, S. R. (2006). The consequences of childhood overweight and obesity. *The Future of Children, 16*(1), 47–67. https://doi.org/10.1353/foc.2006.0004

Darling, K. E., & Sato, A. F. (2017). Systematic review and meta-analysis examining the effectiveness of mobile health technologies in using self-monitoring for pediatric weight management. *Childhood Obesity, 13*(5), 347–355. https://doi.org/10.1089/chi.2017.0038

Dassie, F., Favaretto, F., Bettini, S., Parolin, M., Valenti, M., Reschke, F., Danne, T., Vettor, R., Milan, G., & Maffei, P. (2021). Alström syndrome: An ultra-rare monogenic disorder as a model for insulin resistance, type 2 diabetes mellitus and obesity. *Endocrine, 71*(3), 618–625. https://doi.org/10.1007/s12020-021-02643-y

David-Ferdon, C., Vivolo-Kantor, A. M., Dahlberg, L. L., Marshall, K. J., Rainford, N., & Hall, J. E. (2016). *Youth violence prevention: Resource for action.* National Center for Injury Prevention and Control, Centers for Disease Control and Prevention. https://www.cdc.gov/violenceprevention/pdf/YV-Prevention-Resource_508.pdf

Davidson, J. R. (2010). Major depressive disorder treatment guidelines in America and Europe. *The Journal of Clinical Psychiatry, 71*(Suppl. E1), e04. https://doi.org/10.4088/JCP.9058se1c.04gry

Davis, A. M., James, R. L., Boles, R. E., Goetz, J. R., Belmont, J., & Malone, B. (2011). The use of TeleMedicine in the treatment of paediatric obesity: Feasibility and acceptability. *Maternal and Child Nutrition, 7*(1), 71–79. https://doi.org/10.1111/j.1740-8709.2010.00248.x

Davis, A. M., Sampilo, M., Gallagher, K. S., Landrum, Y., & Malone, B. (2013). Treating rural pediatric obesity through telemedicine: Outcomes from a small randomized controlled trial. *Journal of Pediatric Psychology, 38*(9), 932–943. https://doi.org/10.1093/jpepsy/jst005

Davis, J. N., Gunderson, E. P., Gyllenhammer, L. E., & Goran, M. I. (2013). Impact of gestational diabetes mellitus on pubertal changes in adiposity and metabolic profiles in Latino offspring. *The Journal of Pediatrics, 162*(4), 741–745. https://doi.org/10.1016/j.jpeds.2012.10.001

Davison, K. K., Jurkowski, J. M., & Lawson, H. A. (2013). Reframing family-centred obesity prevention using the Family Ecological Model. *Public Health Nutrition, 16*(10), 1861–1869. https://doi.org/10.1017/S1368980012004533

De, S., Small, J., & Baur, L. A. (2008). Overweight and obesity among children with developmental disabilities. *Journal of Intellectual & Developmental Disability, 33*(1), 43–47. https://doi.org/10.1080/13668250701875137

Decaluwé, V., & Braet, C. (2004). Assessment of eating disorder psychopathology in obese children and adolescents: Interview versus self-report questionnaire. *Behaviour Research and Therapy, 42*(7), 799–811. https://doi.org/10.1016/j.brat.2003.07.008

Decker, K. M., Reiter-Purtill, J., Bejarano, C. M., Goldschmidt, A. B., Mitchell, J. E., Jenkins, T. M., Helmrath, M., Inge, T. H., Michalsky, M. P., & Zeller, M. H. (2022). Psychosocial predictors of problematic eating in young adults who underwent adolescent bariatric surgery. *Obesity Science and Practice, 8*(5), 545–555. https://doi.org/10.1002/osp4.590

Deforche, B., De Bourdeaudhuij, I., Debode, P., Vinaimont, F., Hills, A. P., Verstraete, S., & Bouckaert, J. (2003). Changes in fat mass, fat-free mass and aerobic fitness in severely obese children and adolescents following a residential treatment programme. *European Journal of Pediatrics, 162*(9), 616–622. https://doi.org/10.1007/s00431-003-1247-2

Delaney, C. B., Eddy, K. T., Hartmann, A. S., Becker, A. E., Murray, H. B., & Thomas, J. J. (2015). Pica and rumination behavior among individuals seeking treatment for eating disorders or obesity. *International Journal of Eating Disorders, 48*(2), 238–248. https://doi.org/10.1002/eat.22279

Dennis, K., Le Grange, D., & Bremer, J. (2006). Olanzapine use in adolescent anorexia nervosa. *Eating and Weight Disorders, 11*(2), e53–e56. https://doi.org/10.1007/BF03327760

Dietz, W. H., Baur, L. A., Hall, K., Puhl, R. M., Taveras, E. M., Uauy, R., & Kopelman, P. (2015). Management of obesity: Improvement of health-care training and systems for prevention and care. *The Lancet, 385*(9986), 2521–2533. https://doi.org/10.1016/S0140-6736(14)61748-7

Dimitropoulos, G., Kimber, M., Singh, M., Williams, E. P., Loeb, K. L., Hughes, E. K., Garber, A., Elliott, A., Vyver, E., & Le Grange, D. (2019). Stay the course: Practitioner reflections on implementing family-based treatment with adolescents with atypical anorexia. *Journal of Eating Disorders, 7*(1), 10. https://doi.org/10.1186/s40337-019-0240-8

Dold, M., Aigner, M., Klabunde, M., Treasure, J., & Kasper, S. (2015). Second-generation antipsychotic drugs in anorexia nervosa: A meta-analysis of randomized controlled trials. *Psychotherapy and Psychosomatics, 84*(2), 110–116. https://doi.org/10.1159/000369978

Domoff, S. E., & Niec, L. N. (2018). Parent–child interaction therapy as a prevention model for childhood obesity: A novel application for high-risk families. *Children and Youth Services Review, 91*, 77–84. https://doi.org/10.1016/j.childyouth.2018.05.024

Donaldson, E. A., Cohen, J. E., Villanti, A. C., Kanarek, N. F., Barry, C. L., & Rutkow, L. (2015). Patterns and predictors of state adult obesity prevention legislation enactment in US states: 2010–2013. *Preventive Medicine, 74*, 117–122. https://doi.org/10.1016/j.ypmed.2015.02.013

Döring, N., Ghaderi, A., Bohman, B., Heitmann, B. L., Larsson, C., Berglind, D., Hansson, L., Sundblom, E., Magnusson, M., Blennow, M., Tynelius, P., Forsberg, L., & Rasmussen, F. (2016). Motivational interviewing to prevent childhood obesity: A cluster RCT. *Pediatrics, 137*(5), e20153104. https://doi.org/10.1542/peds.2015-3104

Drucker, D. J. (2022). GLP-1 physiology informs the pharmacotherapy of obesity. *Molecular Metabolism, 57*, 101351. https://doi.org/10.1016/j.molmet.2021.101351

Du, Z. Q., Li, J. J., Huang, J. A., Ma, J., Xu, X. Y., Zou, R., & Xu, X. (2021). Executive functions in predicting weight loss and obesity indicators: A meta-analysis. *Frontiers in Psychology, 11*, 604113. https://doi.org/10.3389/fpsyg.2020.604113

Duncan, A. E., Ziobrowski, H. N., & Nicol, G. (2017). The prevalence of past 12-month and lifetime *DSM-IV* eating disorders by BMI category in US men and women. *European Eating Disorders Review, 25*(3), 165–171. https://doi.org/10.1002/erv.2503

Efe, Y. S., Özbey, H., Erdem, E., & Hatipoğlu, N. (2020). A comparison of emotional eating, social anxiety and parental attitude among adolescents with obesity and healthy: A case-control study. *Archives of Psychiatric Nursing, 34*(6), 557–562. https://doi.org/10.1016/j.apnu.2020.09.007

Egede, L. E., Campbell, J. A., Walker, R. J., & Linde, S. (2023). Structural racism as an upstream social determinant of diabetes outcomes: A scoping review. *Diabetes Care, 46*(4), 667–677. https://doi.org/10.2337/dci22-0044

Eiffener, E., Eli, K., Ek, A., Sandvik, P., Somaraki, M., Kremers, S., Sleddens, E., & Nowicka, P. (2019). The influence of preschoolers' emotional and behavioural problems on obesity treatment outcomes: Secondary findings from a randomized controlled trial. *Pediatric Obesity, 14*(11), e12556. https://doi.org/10.1111/ijpo.12556

Eisenberg, M. E., Carlson-McGuire, A., Gollust, S. E., & Neumark-Sztainer, D. (2015). A content analysis of weight stigmatization in popular television programming for adolescents. *International Journal of Eating Disorders, 48*(6), 759–766. https://doi.org/10.1002/eat.22348

Elbel, B., Tamura, K., McDermott, Z. T., Wu, E., & Schwartz, A. E. (2020). Childhood obesity and the food environment: A population-based sample of public school children in New York City. *Obesity, 28*(1), 65–72. https://doi.org/10.1002/oby.22663

Emerson, E. (2009). Overweight and obesity in 3- and 5-year-old children with and without developmental delay. *Public Health, 123*(2), 130–133. https://doi.org/10.1016/j.puhe.2008.10.020

Emmer, C., Bosnjak, M., & Mata, J. (2020). The association between weight stigma and mental health: A meta-analysis. *Obesity Reviews, 21*(1), e12935. https://doi.org/10.1111/obr.12935

Epstein, L. H., Paluch, R. A., Kilanowski, C. K., & Raynor, H. A. (2004). The effect of reinforcement or stimulus control to reduce sedentary behavior in the treatment of pediatric obesity. *Health Psychology, 23*(4), 371–380. https://doi.org/10.1037/0278-6133.23.4.371

Epstein, L. H., & Squires, S. (1988). *The Stoplight Diet for children: An eight-week program for parents and children.* University of Pittsburgh.

Esani, M. (2016). *Predictors and outcomes of pica* [Unpublished doctoral dissertation]. The University of Texas Medical Branch.

Expert Panel on Integrated Guidelines for Cardiovascular Health and Risk Reduction in Children and Adolescents & National Heart, Lung, and Blood Institute. (2011). Expert Panel on Integrated Guidelines for Cardiovascular Health and Risk Reduction in Children and Adolescents: Summary report. *Pediatrics, 128*(Suppl. 5), S213–S256. https://doi.org/10.1542/peds.2009-2107C

Eyberg, S., & Funderburk, B. (2011). *Parent–Child Interaction Therapy Protocol.* PCIT International.

Fabiano, G. A., Schatz, N. K., & Pelham, W. E., Jr. (2014). Summer treatment programs for youth with ADHD. *Child and Adolescent Psychiatric Clinics of North America, 23*(4), 757–773. https://doi.org/10.1016/j.chc.2014.05.012

Fairburn, C. G., Cooper, Z., & Shafran, R. (2003). Cognitive behaviour therapy for eating disorders: A "transdiagnostic" theory and treatment. *Behaviour Research and Therapy, 41*(5), 509–528. https://doi.org/10.1016/S0005-7967(02)00088-8

Favieri, F., Forte, G., & Casagrande, M. (2019). The executive functions in overweight and obesity: A systematic review of neuropsychological cross-sectional and longitudinal studies. *Frontiers in Psychology, 10,* 2126. https://doi.org/10.3389/fpsyg.2019.02126

Field, A. E., Sonneville, K. R., Micali, N., Crosby, R. D., Swanson, S. A., Laird, N. M., Treasure, J., Solmi, F., & Horton, N. J. (2012). Prospective association of common eating disorders and adverse outcomes. *Pediatrics, 130*(2), e289–e295. https://doi.org/10.1542/peds.2011-3663

Fields, L. C., Brown, C., Skelton, J. A., Cain, K. S., & Cohen, G. M. (2021). Internalized weight bias, teasing, and self-esteem in children with overweight or obesity. *Childhood Obesity, 17*(1), 43–50. https://doi.org/10.1089/chi.2020.0150

Findholt, N. E., Davis, M. M., & Michael, Y. L. (2013). Perceived barriers, resources, and training needs of rural primary care providers relevant to the management of childhood obesity. *The Journal of Rural Health, 29*(Suppl. 1), s17–s24. https://doi.org/10.1111/jrh.12006

Finkelstein, E. A., Trogdon, J. G., Cohen, J. W., & Dietz, W. (2009). Annual medical spending attributable to obesity: Payer- and service-specific estimates. *Health Affairs, 28*(5, Suppl. 1), w822–w831. https://doi.org/10.1377/hlthaff.28.5.w822

Fisch, C., Whelan, J., Evans, S., Whitaker, L. A., Gajjar, S., Ali, L., Fugate, C., Puhl, R., & Hartwell, M. (2022). Use of person-centred language among scientific research focused on childhood obesity. *Pediatric Obesity, 17*(5), e12879. https://doi.org/10.1111/ijpo.12879

Fisher, J. O., & Kral, T. V. (2008). Super-size me: Portion size effects on young children's eating. *Physiology & Behavior, 94*(1), 39–47. https://doi.org/10.1016/j.physbeh.2007.11.015

Fisher, W. W., Piazza, C. C., & Roane, H. S. (2021). *Handbook of applied behavior analysis* (2nd ed.). Guilford Press.

FitzGerald, C., & Hurst, S. (2017). Implicit bias in healthcare professionals: A systematic review. *BMC Medical Ethics, 18*(1), 19. https://doi.org/10.1186/s12910-017-0179-8

Fitzgerald, D. A., Nunn, K., & Isaacs, D. (2021). What we have learnt about trauma, loss and grief for children in response to COVID-19. *Paediatric Respiratory Reviews, 39,* 16–21. https://doi.org/10.1016/j.prrv.2021.05.009

Flodgren, G. M., Helleve, A., Lobstein, T., Rutter, H., & Klepp, K. I. (2020). Primary prevention of overweight and obesity in adolescents: An overview of systematic reviews. *Obesity Reviews, 21*(11), e13102. https://doi.org/10.1111/obr.13102

Fong, V., & Iarocci, G. (2020). Child and family outcomes following pandemics: A systematic review and recommendations on COVID-19 policies. *Journal of Pediatric Psychology, 45*(10), 1124–1143. https://doi.org/10.1093/jpepsy/jsaa092

Fornari, E., Brusati, M., & Maffeis, C. (2021). Nutritional strategies for childhood obesity prevention. *Life, 11*(6), 532. https://doi.org/10.3390/life11060532

Forsythe, E., & Beales, P. L. (2013). Bardet–Biedl syndrome. *European Journal of Human Genetics, 21*(1), 8–13. https://doi.org/10.1038/ejhg.2012.115

Fox, C. L., & Boulton, M. J. (2005). The social skills problems of victims of bullying: Self, peer and teacher perceptions. *British Journal of Educational Psychology, 75*(2), 313–328. https://doi.org/10.1348/000709905X25517

Fradkin, C., Wallander, J. L., Elliott, M. N., Tortolero, S., Cuccaro, P., & Schuster, M. A. (2015). Associations between socioeconomic status and obesity in diverse, young adolescents: Variation across race/ethnicity and gender. *Health Psychology, 34*(1), 1–9. https://doi.org/10.1037/hea0000099

Franckle, R., Adler, R., & Davison, K. (2014). Accelerated weight gain among children during summer versus school year and related racial/ethnic disparities: A systematic review. *Preventing Chronic Disease, 11*, 130355. https://doi.org/10.5888/pcd11.130355

Franklin, J., Denyer, G., Steinbeck, K. S., Caterson, I. D., & Hill, A. J. (2006). Obesity and risk of low self-esteem: A statewide survey of Australian children. *Pediatrics, 118*(6), 2481–2487. https://doi.org/10.1542/peds.2006-0511

Freedman, D. S., Wang, J., Thornton, J. C., Mei, Z., Pierson, R. N., Jr., Dietz, W. H., & Horlick, M. (2008). Racial/ethnic differences in body fatness among children and adolescents. *Obesity, 16*(5), 1105–1111. https://doi.org/10.1038/oby.2008.30

Freizinger, M., Recto, M., Jhe, G., & Lin, J. (2022). Atypical anorexia in youth: Cautiously bridging the treatment gap. *Children, 9*(6), 837. https://doi.org/10.3390/children9060837

Frongillo, E. A., Fawcett, S. B., Ritchie, L. D., Sonia Arteaga, S., Loria, C. M., Pate, R. R., John, L. V., Strauss, W. J., Gregoriou, M., Collie-Akers, V. L., Schultz, J. A., Landgraf, A. J., & Nagaraja, J. (2017). Community policies and programs to prevent obesity and child adiposity. *American Journal of Preventive Medicine, 53*(5), 576–583. https://doi.org/10.1016/j.amepre.2017.05.006

Fryar, C. D., Carroll, M. D., & Afful, J. (2020). *Prevalence of overweight, obesity, and severe obesity among adults aged 20 and over: United States, 1960–1962 through 2017–2018*. National Center for Health Statistics. https://www.cdc.gov/nchs/data/hestat/obesity-adult-17-18/obesity-adult.htm

Gagne, J. R., Liew, J., & Nwadinobi, O. K. (2021). How does the broader construct of self-regulation relate to emotion regulation in young children? *Developmental Review, 60*, 100965. https://doi.org/10.1016/j.dr.2021.100965

Galmiche, M., Déchelotte, P., Lambert, G., & Tavolacci, M. P. (2019). Prevalence of eating disorders over the 2000–2018 period: A systematic literature review. *The American Journal of Clinical Nutrition, 109*(5), 1402–1413. https://doi.org/10.1093/ajcn/nqy342

Garber, A. K. (2018). Moving beyond "skinniness": Presentation weight is not sufficient to assess malnutrition in patients with restrictive eating disorders across a range of body weights. *Journal of Adolescent Health, 63*(6), 669–670. https://doi.org/10.1016/j.jadohealth.2018.09.010

Garland, E., Kutcher, S., Virani, A., & Elbe, D. (2016). Update on the use of SSRIs and SNRIs with children and adolescents in clinical practice. *Journal of the Canadian Academy of Child and Adolescent Psychiatry, 25*(1), 4–10.

Gately, P. J., Cooke, C. B., Barth, J. H., Bewick, B. M., Radley, D., & Hill, A. J. (2005). Children's residential weight-loss programs can work: A prospective cohort study of short-term outcomes for overweight and obese children. *Pediatrics, 116*(1), 73–77. https://doi.org/10.1542/peds.2004-0397

Gately, P. J., Cooke, C. B., Butterly, R. J., Knight, C., & Carroll, S. (2000). The acute effects of an 8-week diet, exercise, and educational camp program on obese children. *Pediatric Exercise Science, 12*(4), 413–423. https://doi.org/10.1123/pes.12.4.413

Germann, J. N., Kirschenbaum, D. S., & Rich, B. H. (2007). Child and parental self-monitoring as determinants of success in the treatment of morbid obesity in low-income minority children. *Journal of Pediatric Psychology, 32*(1), 111–121. https://doi.org/10.1093/jpepsy/jsl007

Gianini, L. M., White, M. A., & Masheb, R. M. (2013). Eating pathology, emotion regulation, and emotional overeating in obese adults with binge eating disorder. *Eating Behaviors, 14*(3), 309–313. https://doi.org/10.1016/j.eatbeh.2013.05.008

Gibson, L. Y., Allen, K. L., Davis, E., Blair, E., Zubrick, S. R., & Byrne, S. M. (2017). The psychosocial burden of childhood overweight and obesity: Evidence for persisting difficulties in boys and girls. *European Journal of Pediatrics, 176*(7), 925–933. https://doi.org/10.1007/s00431-017-2931-y

Gibson, L. Y., Byrne, S. M., Blair, E., Davis, E. A., Jacoby, P., & Zubrick, S. R. (2008). Clustering of psychosocial symptoms in overweight children. *Australian & New Zealand Journal of Psychiatry, 42*(2), 118–125. https://doi.org/10.1080/00048670701787560

Girela-Serrano, B. M., Spiers, A. D. V., Ruotong, L., Gangadia, S., Toledano, M. B., & Di Simplicio, M. (2022). Impact of mobile phones and wireless devices use on children and adolescents' mental health: A systematic review. *European Child & Adolescent Psychiatry*, 1–31. https://doi.org/10.1007/s00787-022-02012-8

Global Weight Loss Products and Services Market Report 2021: The business of weight loss in the 20th and 21st centuries. (2021, August 13). https://www.prnewswire.com/news-releases/global-weight-loss-products-and-services-market-report-2021-the-business-of-weight-loss-in-the-20th-and-21st-centuries-301354957.html#:~:text=The%20global%20market%20for%20weight, forecast%20period%20of%202021%2D2026

Golan, M. (2006). Parents as agents of change in childhood obesity—From research to practice. *International Journal of Pediatric Obesity, 1*(2), 66–76. https://doi.org/10.1080/17477160600644272

Golden, N. H., Schneider, M., Wood, C., Committee on Nutrition, Committee on Adolescence, Section on Obesity, Daniels, S., Abrams, S., Corkins, M., de Ferranti, S., Magge, S. N., Schwarzenberg, S., Braverman, P. K., Adelman, W., Alderman, E. M., Breuner, C. C., Levine, D. A., Marcell, A. V., O'Brien, R., . . . Slusser, W. (2016). Preventing obesity and eating disorders in adolescents. *Pediatrics, 138*(3), e20161649. https://doi.org/10.1542/peds.2016-1649

Goldstein, B. I., Birmaher, B., Axelson, D. A., Goldstein, T. R., Esposito-Smythers, C., Strober, M. A., Hunt, J., Leonard, H., Gill, M. K., Iyengar, S., Grimm, C., Yang, M., Ryan, N. D., & Keller, M. B. (2008). Preliminary findings regarding overweight and obesity in pediatric bipolar disorder. *The Journal of Clinical Psychiatry, 69*(12), 1953–1959. https://doi.org/10.4088/JCP.v69n1215

Goldstein, S. P., Goldstein, C. M., Bond, D. S., Raynor, H. A., Wing, R. R., & Thomas, J. G. (2019). Associations between self-monitoring and weight change in behavioral weight loss interventions. *Health Psychology, 38*(12), 1128–1136. https://doi.org/10.1037/hea0000800

Gómez, C. A., Kleinman, D. V., Pronk, N., Gordon, G. L. W., Ochiai, E., Blakey, C., Johnson, A., & Brewer, K. H. (2021). Practice full report: Addressing health equity and social determinants of health through Healthy People 2030. *Journal of Public Health Management and Practice, 27*(6), S249–S257. https://doi.org/10.1097/PHH.0000000000001297

Goodman, E., & Whitaker, R. C. (2002). A prospective study of the role of depression in the development and persistence of adolescent obesity. *Pediatrics, 110*(3), 497–504. https://doi.org/10.1542/peds.110.3.497

Goodman, M., Thomson, J., & Landry, A. (2020). Food environment in the lower Mississippi Delta: Food deserts, food swamps and hot spots. *International Journal of Environmental Research and Public Health, 17*(10), 3354. https://doi.org/10.3390/ijerph17103354

Goodman, R. (1997). The Strengths and Difficulties Questionnaire: A research note. *Journal of Child Psychology and Psychiatry, 38*(5), 581–586. https://doi.org/10.1111/j.1469-7610.1997.tb01545.x

Gorlick, J. C., Gorman, C. V., Weeks, H. M., Pearlman, A. T., Schvey, N. A., & Bauer, K. W. (2021). "I feel like less of a mom": Experiences of weight stigma by association among mothers of children with overweight and obesity. *Childhood Obesity, 17*(1), 68–75. https://doi.org/10.1089/chi.2020.0199

Gourlan, M., Sarrazin, P., & Trouilloud, D. (2013). Motivational interviewing as a way to promote physical activity in obese adolescents: A randomised-controlled trial using self-determination theory as an explanatory framework.

Psychology & Health, 28(11), 1265–1286. https://doi.org/10.1080/08870446. 2013.800518

Gowey, M. A., Lim, C. S., Dutton, G. R., Silverstein, J. H., Dumont-Driscoll, M. C., & Janicke, D. M. (2018). Executive function and dysregulated eating behaviors in pediatric obesity. *Journal of Pediatric Psychology, 43*(8), 834–845. https://doi.org/10.1093/jpepsy/jsx091

Gowey, M. A., Neumeier, W. H., Henry, S., Wadley, V. G., Phillips, J., Hayden, K. M., Espeland, M. A., Coday, M., Lewis, C. E., & Dutton, G. R. (2021). Executive function in individuals with clinically significant weight loss via behavioral intervention. *Obesity Science & Practice, 7*(1), 25–34. https://doi.org/10.1002/osp4.458

Gowey, M., Redden, D., Lim, C., Janicke, D., & Dutton, G. (2020). Executive function phenotypes in pediatric obesity. *Pediatric Obesity, 15*(9), e12655. https://doi.org/10.1111/ijpo.12655

Gowey, M. A., Stromberg, S., Lim, C. S., & Janicke, D. M. (2017). The moderating role of body dissatisfaction in the relationship between ADHD symptoms and disordered eating in pediatric overweight and obesity. *Children's Health Care, 46*(1), 15–33. https://doi.org/10.1080/02739615.2015.1065745

Graber, J. A. (2004). Internalizing problems during adolescence. In R. M. Lerner & L. Steinberg (Eds.), *Handbook of adolescent psychology* (pp. 587–626). Wiley.

Graham, C., & Frisco, M. (2022). The relationship between obesity and suicide ideation among young adults in the United States. *SSM—Population Health, 18*, 101106. https://doi.org/10.1016/j.ssmph.2022.101106

Grammer, A. C., Tanofsky-Kraff, M., Burke, N. L., Byrne, M. E., Mi, S. J., Jaramillo, M., Shank, L. M., Kelly, N. R., Stojek, M. M., Schvey, N. A., Broadney, M. M., Brady, S. M., Yanovski, S. Z., & Yanovski, J. A. (2018). An examination of the associations between pediatric loss of control eating, anxiety, and body composition in children and adolescents. *Eating Behaviors, 30*, 109–114. https://doi.org/10.1016/j.eatbeh.2018.06.007

Gray, E. W., Smith, W. A., Burton, E. T., Hale, D., Odulana, A., & Weatherall, Y. Z. (2023). Insurance approval for laparoscopic sleeve gastrectomy in adolescents in the Midsouth. *Childhood Obesity.* Advance online publication. https://doi.org/10.1089/chi.2022.0175

Graziano, P. A., Bagner, D. M., Waxmonsky, J. G., Reid, A., McNamara, J. P., & Geffken, G. R. (2012). Co-occurring weight problems among children with attention deficit/hyperactivity disorder: The role of executive functioning. *International Journal of Obesity, 36*(4), 567–572. https://doi.org/10.1038/ijo.2011.245

Graziano, P. A., Calkins, S. D., & Keane, S. P. (2010). Toddler self-regulation skills predict risk for pediatric obesity. *International Journal of Obesity, 34*(4), 633–641. https://doi.org/10.1038/ijo.2009.288

Graziano, P. A., Garcia, A., & Lim, C. S. (2017). Summer Healthy-Lifestyle Intervention Program for young children who are overweight: Results from a nonrandomized pilot trial. *Journal of Developmental & Behavioral Pediatrics, 38*(9), 723–727. https://doi.org/10.1097/DBP.0000000000000499

Graziano, P. A., Kelleher, R., Calkins, S. D., Keane, S. P., & Brien, M. O. (2013). Predicting weight outcomes in preadolescence: The role of toddlers' self-regulation skills and the temperament dimension of pleasure. *International Journal of Obesity, 37*(7), 937–942. https://doi.org/10.1038/ijo.2012.165

Greenberg, J. A. (2013). Obesity and early mortality in the United States. *Obesity, 21*(2), 405–412. https://doi.org/10.1002/oby.20023

Greenleaf, C., Martin, S. B., & Rhea, D. (2008). Fighting fat: How do fat stereotypes influence beliefs about physical education? *Obesity, 16*(Suppl. 2), S53–S59. https://doi.org/10.1038/oby.2008.454

Greenway, F. L. (2015). Physiological adaptations to weight loss and factors favouring weight regain. *International Journal of Obesity, 39*(8), 1188–1196. https://doi.org/10.1038/ijo.2015.59

Grilo, C. M. (2013). Why no cognitive body image feature such as overvaluation of shape/weight in the binge eating disorder diagnosis? *International Journal of Eating Disorders, 46*(3), 208–211. https://doi.org/10.1002/eat.22082

Grilo, C. M., White, M. A., & Masheb, R. M. (2009). *DSM-IV* psychiatric disorder comorbidity and its correlates in binge eating disorder. *International Journal of Eating Disorders, 42*(3), 228–234. https://doi.org/10.1002/eat.20599

Guedj, R., Marini, M., Kossowsky, J., Berde, C., Mateo, C., & Fleegler, E. W. (2021). Explicit and implicit bias based on race, ethnicity, and weight among pediatric emergency physicians. *Academic Emergency Medicine, 28*(9), 1073–1076. https://doi.org/10.1111/acem.14301

Gulati, A. K., Kaplan, D. W., & Daniels, S. R. (2012). Clinical tracking of severely obese children: A new growth chart. *Pediatrics, 130*(6), 1136–1140. https://doi.org/10.1542/peds.2012-0596

Gunderson, E. P., Greenspan, L. C., Faith, M. S., Hurston, S. R., Quesenberry, C. P., Jr., & SWIFT Offspring Study Investigators. (2018). Breastfeeding and growth during infancy among offspring of mothers with gestational diabetes mellitus: A prospective cohort study. *Pediatric Obesity, 13*(8), 492–504.

Gunstad, J., Sanborn, V., & Hawkins, M. (2020). Cognitive dysfunction is a risk factor for overeating and obesity. *American Psychologist, 75*(2), 219–234. https://doi.org/10.1037/amp0000585

Gutierrez-Colina, A. M., Clifford, L., Wade, S. L., & Modi, A. C. (2022). Uncovering key elements of an executive functioning intervention in adolescents: Epilepsy journey. *Clinical Practice in Pediatric Psychology, 10*(2), 150–163. https://doi.org/10.1037/cpp0000410

Haines, J., Neumark-Sztainer, D., Eisenberg, M. E., & Hannan, P. J. (2006). Weight teasing and disordered eating behaviors in adolescents: Longitudinal findings from Project EAT (Eating Among Teens). *Pediatrics, 117*(2), e209–e215. https://doi.org/10.1542/peds.2005-1242

Hales, C. M., Carroll, M. D., Fryar, C. D., & Ogden, C. L. (2017, October). *Prevalence of obesity among adults and youth: United States, 2015–2016.* NCHS Data Brief No. 288. https://www.cdc.gov/nchs/data/databriefs/db288.pdf

Hales, C. M., Carroll, M. D., Fryar, C. D., & Ogden, C. L. (2020, February). *Prevalence of obesity and severe obesity among adults: United States, 2017–2018.*

NCHS Data Brief No. 360. https://www.cdc.gov/nchs/products/databriefs/db360.htm

Hales, C. M., Freedman, D. S., Akinbami, L., Wei, R., & Ogden, C. L. (2022). Evaluation of alternative body mass index (BMI) metrics to monitor weight status in children and adolescents with extremely high BMI using CDC BMI-for-age growth charts. *Vital and Health Statistics. Ser. 1, Programs and Collection Procedures*, (197), 1–42.

Hall, K. D., Farooqi, I. S., Friedman, J. M., Klein, S., Loos, R. J. F., Mangelsdorf, D. J., O'Rahilly, S., Ravussin, E., Redman, L. M., Ryan, D. H., Speakman, J. R., & Tobias, D. K. (2022). The energy balance model of obesity: Beyond calories in, calories out. *The American Journal of Clinical Nutrition*, *115*(5), 1243–1254. https://doi.org/10.1093/ajcn/nqac031

Hall, K. D., & Guo, J. (2017). Obesity energetics: Body weight regulation and the effects of diet composition. *Gastroenterology*, *152*(7), P1718–P1727.E3. https://doi.org/10.1053/j.gastro.2017.01.052

Hammerle, F., Huss, M., Ernst, V., & Bürger, A. (2016). Thinking dimensional: Prevalence of *DSM-5* early adolescent full syndrome, partial and subthreshold eating disorders in a cross-sectional survey in German schools. *BMJ Open*, *6*(5), e010843. https://doi.org/10.1136/bmjopen-2015-010843

Hampl, S. E., Hassink, S. G., Skinner, A. C., Armstrong, S. C., Barlow, S. E., Bolling, C. F., Avila Edwards, K. C., Eneli, I., Hamre, R., Joseph, M. M., Lunsford, D., Mendonca, E., Michalsky, M. P., Mirza, N., Ochoa, E. R., Jr., Sharifi, M., Staiano, A. E., Weedn, A. E., Flinn, S. K., . . . Okechukwu, K. (2023a). Clinical practice guideline for the evaluation and treatment of children and adolescents with obesity. *Pediatrics*, *151*(2), e2022060640. https://doi.org/10.1542/peds.2022-060640

Hampl, S. E., Hassink, S. G., Skinner, A. C., Armstrong, S. C., Barlow, S. E., Bolling, C. F., Avila Edwards, K. C., Eneli, I., Hamre, R., Joseph, M. M., Lunsford, D., Mendonca, E., Michalsky, M. P., Mirza, N., Ochoa, E. R., Jr., Sharifi, M., Staiano, A. E., Weedn, A. E., Flinn, S. K., . . . Okechukwu, K. (2023b). Executive summary: Clinical practice guideline for the evaluation and treatment of children and adolescents with obesity. *Pediatrics*, *151*(2), e2022060641. https://doi.org/10.1542/peds.2022-060641

Haqq, A. M., Kebbe, M., Tan, Q., Manco, M., & Salas, X. R. (2021). Complexity and stigma of pediatric obesity. *Childhood Obesity*, *17*(4), 229–240. https://doi.org/10.1089/chi.2021.0003

Hardy, L. L., Booth, M. L., & Okely, A. D. (2007). The reliability of the Adolescent Sedentary Activity Questionnaire (ASAQ). *Preventive Medicine*, *45*(1), 71–74. https://doi.org/10.1016/j.ypmed.2007.03.014

Harriger, J. A., & Thompson, J. K. (2012). Psychological consequences of obesity: Weight bias and body image in overweight and obese youth. *International Review of Psychiatry*, *24*(3), 247–253. https://doi.org/10.3109/09540261.2012.678817

Harris, E. (2023). Triple-hormone combination retatrutide induces 24% body weight loss. *JAMA, 30*(4), 306. https://doi.org/10.1001/jama.2023.12055

Harrop, E. N., Mensinger, J. L., Moore, M., & Lindhorst, T. (2021). Restrictive eating disorders in higher weight persons: A systematic review of atypical anorexia nervosa prevalence and consecutive admission literature. *International Journal of Eating Disorders, 54*(8), 1328–1357. https://doi.org/10.1002/eat.23519

Harshman, S. G., Wons, O., Rogers, M. S., Izquierdo, A. M., Holmes, T. M., Pulumo, R. L., Asanza, E., Eddy, K. T., Misra, M., Micali, N., Lawson, E. A., & Thomas, J. J. (2019). A diet high in processed foods, total carbohydrates and added sugars, and low in vegetables and protein is characteristic of youth with avoidant/restrictive food intake disorder. *Nutrients, 11*(9), 2013. https://doi.org/10.3390/nu11092013

Hawkes, C., Jewell, J., & Allen, K. (2013). A food policy package for healthy diets and the prevention of obesity and diet-related non-communicable diseases: The NOURISHING framework. *Obesity Reviews, 14*(Suppl. 2), 159–168. https://doi.org/10.1111/obr.12098

Hayes, J. F., Fitzsimmons-Craft, E. E., Karam, A. M., Jakubiak, J., Brown, M. L., & Wilfley, D. E. (2018). Disordered eating attitudes and behaviors in youth with overweight and obesity: Implications for treatment. *Current Obesity Reports, 7*(3), 235–246. https://doi.org/10.1007/s13679-018-0316-9

Hayes, S. C., & Hofmann, S. G. (2017). The third wave of cognitive behavioral therapy and the rise of process-based care. *World Psychiatry, 16*(3), 245–246. https://doi.org/10.1002/wps.20442

Healy, S., Aigner, C. J., & Haegele, J. A. (2019). Prevalence of overweight and obesity among US youth with autism spectrum disorder. *Autism, 23*(4), 1046–1050. https://doi.org/10.1177/1362361318791817

Hedegaard, H., Curtin, S. C., & Warner, M. (2021, February). *Suicide mortality in the United States, 1999–2019.* NCHS Data Brief No. 398. https://www.cdc.gov/nchs/products/databriefs/db398.htm

Heindel, J. J., & Blumberg, B. (2019). Environmental obesogens: Mechanisms and controversies. *Annual Review of Pharmacology and Toxicology, 59*, 89–106. https://doi.org/10.1146/annurev-pharmtox-010818-021304

Hembree-Kigin, T. L., & McNeil, C. B. (1995). *Parent–child interaction therapy.* Kluwer Academic/Plenum Press. https://doi.org/10.1007/978-1-4899-1439-2

Hemmingsson, E. (2018). Early childhood obesity risk factors: Socioeconomic adversity, family dysfunction, offspring distress, and junk food self-medication. *Current Obesity Reports, 7*(2), 204–209. https://doi.org/10.1007/s13679-018-0310-2

Hendricks, E. J., Srisurapanont, M., Schmidt, S. L., Haggard, M., Souter, S., Mitchell, C. L., De Marco, D. G., Hendricks, M. J., Istratiy, Y., & Greenway, F. L. (2014). Addiction potential of phentermine prescribed during long-term treatment of obesity. *International Journal of Obesity, 38*(2), 292–298. https://doi.org/10.1038/ijo.2013.74

Hennessy, E., Hughes, S. O., Goldberg, J. P., Hyatt, R. R., & Economos, C. D. (2010). Parent–child interactions and objectively measured child physical activity: A cross-sectional study. *International Journal of Behavioral Nutrition and Physical Activity, 7*, 1–14. https://doi.org/10.1186/1479-5868-7-71

Herdes, R. E., Tsao, D. D., & Pratt, J. S. A. (2021). Why earlier may be better: A look at the use of metabolic and bariatric surgery in the treatment of severe childhood obesity. *Surgery for Obesity and Related Diseases, 17*(12), 2107–2110. https://doi.org/10.1016/j.soard.2021.09.003

Hilbert, A., Petroff, D., Neuhaus, P., & Schmidt, R. (2020). Cognitive–behavioral therapy for adolescents with an age-adapted diagnosis of binge-eating disorder: A randomized clinical trial. *Psychotherapy and Psychosomatics, 89*(1), 51–53. https://doi.org/10.1159/000503116

Hilbert, A., Ried, J., Schneider, D., Juttner, C., Sosna, M., Dabrock, P., Lingenfelder, M., Voit, W., Rief, W., & Hebebrand, J. (2008). Primary prevention of childhood obesity: An interdisciplinary analysis. *Obesity Facts, 1*(1), 16–25. https://doi.org/10.1159/000113598

Hing, E., & Hsiao, C.-J. (2014, May). *State variability in supply of office-based primary care providers, United States, 2012.* NCHS Data Brief No. 151. https://www.cdc.gov/nchs/products/databriefs/db151.htm

Hinkle, K. A., Kirschenbaum, D. S., Pecora, K. M., & Germann, J. N. (2011). Parents may hold the keys to success in immersion treatment of adolescent obesity. *Child & Family Behavior Therapy, 33*(4), 273–288. https://doi.org/10.1080/07317107.2011.623085

Hoeltzel, G. D., Swendiman, R. A., Tewksbury, C. M., Parks, E. P., Williams, N. N., & Dumon, K. R. (2022). How safe is adolescent bariatric surgery? An analysis of short-term outcomes. *Journal of Pediatric Surgery, 57*(8), 1654–1659. https://doi.org/10.1016/j.jpedsurg.2021.08.018

Hooper, M. W., Nápoles, A. M., & Pérez-Stable, E. J. (2020). COVID-19 and racial/ethnic disparities. *JAMA, 323*(24), 2466–2467. https://doi.org/10.1001/jama.2020.8598

Howard, J. B., Skinner, A. C., Ravanbakht, S. N., Brown, J. D., Perrin, A. J., Steiner, M. J., & Perrin, E. M. (2017). Obesogenic behavior and weight-based stigma in popular children's movies, 2012 to 2015. *Pediatrics, 140*(6), e20172126. https://doi.org/10.1542/peds.2017-2126

Hudson, J. I., Hiripi, E., Pope, H. G., Jr., & Kessler, R. C. (2007). The prevalence and correlates of eating disorders in the National Comorbidity Survey Replication. *Biological Psychiatry, 61*(3), 348–358. https://doi.org/10.1016/j.biopsych.2006.03.040

Huelsing, J., Kanafani, N., Mao, J., & White, N. H. (2010). Camp Jump Start: Effects of a residential summer weight-loss camp for older children and adolescents. *Pediatrics, 125*(4), e884–e890. https://doi.org/10.1542/peds.2009-1007

Hughes, E. K., Le Grange, D., Court, A., & Sawyer, S. M. (2017). A case series of family-based treatment for adolescents with atypical anorexia nervosa.

International Journal of Eating Disorders, *50*(4), 424–432. https://doi.org/10.1002/eat.22662

Hughes, S. O., Power, T. G., Fisher, J. O., Mueller, S., & Nicklas, T. A. (2005). Revisiting a neglected construct: Parenting styles in a child-feeding context. *Appetite*, *44*(1), 83–92. https://doi.org/10.1016/j.appet.2004.08.007

Hughes, S. O., Power, T. G., O'Connor, T. M., & Fisher, J. O. (2015). Executive functioning, emotion regulation, eating self-regulation, and weight status in low-income preschool children: How do they relate? *Appetite*, *89*, 1–9. https://doi.org/10.1016/j.appet.2015.01.009

Hunger, J. M., & Tomiyama, A. J. (2018). Weight labeling and disordered eating among adolescent girls: Longitudinal evidence from the National Heart, Lung, and Blood Institute Growth and Health Study. *Journal of Adolescent Health*, *63*(3), 360–362. https://doi.org/10.1016/j.jadohealth.2017.12.016

Iguacel, I., Gasch-Gallén, Á., Ayala-Marín, A. M., De Miguel-Etayo, P., & Moreno, L. A. (2021). Social vulnerabilities as risk factor of childhood obesity development and their role in prevention programs. *International Journal of Obesity*, *45*(1), 1–11. https://doi.org/10.1038/s41366-020-00697-y

Individuals With Disabilities Education Act of 1990, Pub. L. 101-476, renamed the Individuals With Disabilities Education Improvement Act, codified at 20 U.S.C. §§ 1400–1482.

Infant & Toddler Forum. (2014). *Developmental stages in infant and toddler feeding*. https://infantandtoddlerforum.org/media/upload/pdf-downloads/3.5_Developmental_Stages_in_Infant_and_Toddler_Feeding_NEW.pdf

Inge, T. H., Boyce, T. W., Lee, M., Kollar, L., Jenkins, T. M., Brandt, M. L., Helmrath, M., Xanthakos, S. A., Zeller, M. H., Harmon, C. M., Courcoulas, A., & Michalsky, M. P. (2014). Access to care for adolescents seeking weight loss surgery. *Obesity*, *22*(12), 2593–2597. https://doi.org/10.1002/oby.20898

Inge, T. H., Courcoulas, A. P., Jenkins, T. M., Michalsky, M. P., Brandt, M. L., Xanthakos, S. A., Dixon, J. B., Harmon, C. M., Chen, M. K., Xie, C., Evans, M. E., & Helmrath, M. A. (2019). Five-year outcomes of gastric bypass in adolescents as compared with adults. *The New England Journal of Medicine*, *380*(22), 2136–2145. https://doi.org/10.1056/NEJMoa1813909

Inge, T. H., Courcoulas, A. P., Jenkins, T. M., Michalsky, M. P., Helmrath, M. A., Brandt, M. L., Harmon, C. M., Zeller, M. H., Chen, M. K., Xanthakos, S. A., Horlick, M., & Buncher, C. R. (2016). Weight loss and health status 3 years after bariatric surgery in adolescents. *The New England Journal of Medicine*, *374*(2), 113–123. https://doi.org/10.1056/NEJMoa1506699

Institute of Medicine. (2012). *Accelerating progress in obesity prevention: Solving the weight of the nation*. National Academies Press. https://doi.org/10.17226/13275

Iturbe, I., Echeburúa, E., & Maiz, E. (2022). The effectiveness of acceptance and commitment therapy upon weight management and psychological well-being of adults with overweight or obesity: A systematic review. *Clinical Psychology & Psychotherapy*, *29*(3), 837–856. https://doi.org/10.1002/cpp.2695

Janicke, D. M., Lim, C. S., Mathews, A. E., Shelnutt, K. P., Boggs, S. R., Silverstein, J. H., & Brumback, B. A. (2013). The Community-based Healthy-lifestyle Intervention for Rural Preschools (CHIRP) Study: Design and methods. *Contemporary Clinical Trials, 34*(2), 187–195. https://doi.org/10.1016/j.cct.2012.11.004

Janicke, D. M., Lim, C. S., Perri, M. G., Bobroff, L. B., Mathews, A. E., Brumback, B. A., Dumont-Driscoll, M., & Silverstein, J. H. (2011). The Extension Family Lifestyle Intervention Project (E-FLIP for Kids): Design and methods. *Contemporary Clinical Trials, 32*(1), 50–58. https://doi.org/10.1016/j.cct.2010.08.002

Janicke, D. M., Lim, C. S., Perri, M. G., Mathews, A. E., Bobroff, L. B., Gurka, M. J., Parish, A., Brumback, B. A., Dumont-Driscoll, M., & Silverstein, J. H. (2019). Behavior interventions addressing obesity in rural settings: The E-FLIP for Kids Trial. *Journal of Pediatric Psychology, 44*(8), 889–901. https://doi.org/10.1093/jpepsy/jsz029

Janicke, D. M., Steele, R. G., Gayes, L. A., Lim, C. S., Clifford, L. M., Schneider, E. M., Carmody, J. K., & Westen, S. (2014). Systematic review and meta-analysis of comprehensive behavioral family lifestyle interventions addressing pediatric obesity. *Journal of Pediatric Psychology, 39*(8), 809–825. https://doi.org/10.1093/jpepsy/jsu023

Janssen, I. (2015). Hyper-parenting is negatively associated with physical activity among 7–12 year olds. *Preventive Medicine, 73*, 55–59. https://doi.org/10.1016/j.ypmed.2015.01.015

Jaremka, L. M., & Pacanowski, C. R. (2019). Social anxiety symptoms moderate the link between obesity and metabolic function. *Psychoneuroendocrinology, 110*, 104425. https://doi.org/10.1016/j.psyneuen.2019.104425

Järvholm, K., Karlsson, J., Olbers, T., Peltonen, M., Marcus, C., Dahlgren, J., Gronowitz, E., Johnsson, P., & Flodmark, C.-E. (2016). Characteristics of adolescents with poor mental health after bariatric surgery. *Surgery for Obesity and Related Diseases, 12*(4), 882–890. https://doi.org/10.1016/j.soard.2016.02.001

Jebeile, H., Gow, M. L., Baur, L. A., Garnett, S. P., Paxton, S. J., & Lister, N. B. (2019). Treatment of obesity, with a dietary component, and eating disorder risk in children and adolescents: A systematic review with meta-analysis. *Obesity Reviews, 20*(9), 1287–1298. https://doi.org/10.1111/obr.12866

Jebeile, H., Lister, N. B., Baur, L. A., Garnett, S. P., & Paxton, S. J. (2021). Eating disorder risk in adolescents with obesity. *Obesity Reviews, 22*(5), e13173. https://doi.org/10.1111/obr.13173

Jelalian, E., Jandasek, B., Wolff, J. C., Seaboyer, L. M., Jones, R. N., & Spirito, A. (2019). Cognitive–behavioral therapy plus healthy lifestyle enhancement for depressed, overweight/obese adolescents: Results of a pilot trial. *Journal of Clinical Child and Adolescent Psychology, 48*(Suppl. 1), S24–S33. https://doi.org/10.1080/15374416.2016.1163705

Jelalian, E., Wember, Y. M., Bungeroth, H., & Birmaher, V. (2007). Bridging the gap between research and clinical practice in pediatric obesity. *Journal of Child Psychology and Psychiatry, 48*(2), 115–127. https://doi.org/10.1111/j.1469-7610.2006.01613.x

Jia, P., Xue, H., Cheng, X., Wang, Y., & Wang, Y. (2019). Association of neighborhood built environments with childhood obesity: Evidence from a 9-year longitudinal, nationally representative survey in the US. *Environment International, 128*, 158–164. https://doi.org/10.1016/j.envint.2019.03.067

Johns, M. W. (2015). The assessment of sleepiness in children and adolescents. *Sleep and Biological Rhythms, 13*(Suppl. 1), 97.

Johnson, J. A., III, & Johnson, A. M. (2015). Urban–rural differences in childhood and adolescent obesity in the United States: A systematic review and meta-analysis. *Childhood Obesity, 11*(3), 233–241. https://doi.org/10.1089/chi.2014.0085

Johnson, T. J., Ellison, A. M., Dalembert, G., Fowler, J., Dhingra, M., Shaw, K., & Ibrahim, S. (2017). Implicit bias in pediatric academic medicine. *Journal of the National Medical Association, 109*(3), 156–163. https://doi.org/10.1016/j.jnma.2017.03.003

Johnson, V. R., Cao, M., Czepiel, K. S., Mushannen, T., Nolen, L., & Stanford, F. C. (2020). Strategies in the management of adolescent obesity. *Current Pediatrics Reports, 8*(2), 56–65. https://doi.org/10.1007/s40124-020-00214-9

Johnston, C. A., Moreno, J. P., El-Mubasher, A., Gallagher, M., Tyler, C., & Woehler, D. (2013). Impact of a school-based pediatric obesity prevention program facilitated by health professionals. *Journal of School Health, 83*(3), 171–181. https://doi.org/10.1111/josh.12013

Kalarchian, M. A., & Marcus, M. D. (2012). Psychiatric comorbidity of childhood obesity. *International Review of Psychiatry, 24*(3), 241–246. https://doi.org/10.3109/09540261.2012.678818

Kamody, R. C., Thurston, I. B., & Burton, E. T. (2020). Acceptance-based skill acquisition and cognitive reappraisal in a culturally responsive treatment for binge eating in adolescence. *Eating Disorders, 28*(2), 184–201. https://doi.org/10.1080/10640266.2020.1731055

Kamody, R. C., Thurston, I. B., Decker, K. M., Kaufman, C. C., Sonneville, K. R., & Richmond, T. K. (2018). Relating shape/weight based self-esteem, depression, and anxiety with weight and perceived physical health among young adults. *Body Image, 25*, 168–176. https://doi.org/10.1016/j.bodyim.2018.04.003

Kamody, R. C., Thurston, I. B., Pluhar, E. I., Han, J. C., & Burton, E. T. (2019). Implementing a condensed dialectical behavior therapy skills group for binge-eating behaviors in adolescents. *Eating and Weight Disorders, 24*(2), 367–372. https://doi.org/10.1007/s40519-018-0580-4

Kang, N. R., & Kwack, Y. S. (2020). An update on mental health problems and cognitive behavioral therapy in pediatric obesity. *Pediatric Gastroenterology, Hepatology & Nutrition, 23*(1), 15–25. https://doi.org/10.5223/pghn.2020.23.1.15

Kang, S. (2021). Adipose tissue malfunction drives metabolic dysfunction in Alström syndrome. *Diabetes, 70*(2), 323–325. https://doi.org/10.2337/dbi20-0041

Kaur, H., Li, C., Nazir, N., Choi, W. S., Resnicow, K., Birch, L. L., & Ahluwalia, J. S. (2006). Confirmatory factor analysis of the child-feeding questionnaire among parents of adolescents. *Appetite, 47*(1), 36–45. https://doi.org/10.1016/j.appet.2006.01.020

Kawai, M. (2022). Disruption of the circadian rhythms and its relationship with pediatric obesity. *Pediatrics International, 64*(1), e14992. https://doi.org/10.1111/ped.14992

Keating, S. K., & Wild, C. E. K. (2023). Semaglutide and social media: Implications for young women with polycystic ovarian syndrome. *The Lancet: Child & Adolescent Health, 7*(5), 301–303. https://doi.org/10.1016/S2352-4642(23)00033-0

Kelly, A. S., Fox, C. K., Rudser, K. D., Gross, A. C., & Ryder, J. R. (2016). Pediatric obesity pharmacotherapy: Current state of the field, review of the literature and clinical trial considerations. *International Journal of Obesity, 40*(7), 1043–1050. https://doi.org/10.1038/ijo.2016.69

Kelly, K. P., & Kirschenbaum, D. S. (2011). Immersion treatment of childhood and adolescent obesity: The first review of a promising intervention. *Obesity Reviews, 12*(1), 37–49. https://doi.org/10.1111/j.1467-789X.2009.00710.x

Kennedy, G. A., Forman, S. F., Woods, E. R., Hergenroeder, A. C., Mammel, K. A., Fisher, M. M., Ornstein, R. M., Callahan, S. T., Golden, N. H., Kapphahn, C. J., Garber, A. K., Rome, E. S., & Richmond, T. K. (2017). History of overweight/obesity as predictor of care received at 1-year follow-up in adolescents with anorexia nervosa or atypical anorexia nervosa. *Journal of Adolescent Health, 60*(6), 674–679. https://doi.org/10.1016/j.jadohealth.2017.01.001

Kerem, L., Van De Water, A. L., Kuhnle, M. C., Harshman, S., Hauser, K., Eddy, K. T., Becker, K. R., Misra, M., Macali, N., Thomas, J. J., Holsen, L., & Lawson, E. A. (2022). Neurobiology of avoidant/restrictive food intake disorder in youth with overweight/obesity versus healthy weight. *Journal of Clinical Child & Adolescent Psychology, 51*(5), 701–714. https://doi.org/10.1080/15374416.2021.1894944

Kessler, R. C., Berglund, P. A., Chiu, W. T., Deitz, A. C., Hudson, J. I., Shahly, V., Aguilar-Gaxiola, S., Alonso, J., Angermeyer, M. C., Benjet, C., Bruffaerts, R., de Girolamo, G., de Graaf, R., Maria Haro, J., Kovess-Masfety, V., O'Neill, S., Posada-Villa, J., Sasu, C., Scott, K., . . . Xavier, M. (2013). The prevalence and correlates of binge eating disorder in the World Health Organization World Mental Health Surveys. *Biological Psychiatry, 73*(9), 904–914. https://doi.org/10.1016/j.biopsych.2012.11.020

Khoury, B., Lecomte, T., Fortin, G., Masse, M., Therien, P., Bouchard, V., Chapleau, M. A., Paquin, K., & Hofmann, S. G. (2013). Mindfulness-based therapy: A comprehensive meta-analysis. *Clinical Psychology Review, 33*(6), 763–771. https://doi.org/10.1016/j.cpr.2013.05.005

Kibakaya, E. C., & Oyeku, S. O. (2022). Cultural humility: A critical step in achieving health equity. *Pediatrics, 149*(2), e2021052883. https://doi.org/10.1542/peds.2021-052883

Killion, L., Hughes, S. O., Wendt, J. C., Pease, D., & Nicklas, T. A. (2006). Minority mothers' perceptions of children's body size. *International Journal of Pediatric Obesity, 1*(2), 96–102. https://doi.org/10.1080/17477160600684286

King, K. P., Keller, C. V., Evans, C. T., Murdaugh, D. L., Gower, B. A., & Gowey, M. A. (2023). Inflammation, executive function, and adiposity in children with or at risk for obesity: A pilot study. *Journal of Pediatric Psychology, 48*(2), 134–143. https://doi.org/10.1093/jpepsy/jsac071

Kirk, S., Ogata, B., Wichert, E., Handu, D., & Rozga, M. (2022). Treatment of pediatric overweight and obesity: Position of the Academy of Nutrition and Dietetics based on an umbrella review of systematic reviews. *Journal of the Academy of Nutrition and Dietetics, 122*(4), 848–861. https://doi.org/10.1016/j.jand.2022.01.008

Kirschenbaum, D. S. (2010). Weight-loss camps in the U.S. and the immersion-to-lifestyle change model. *Childhood Obesity, 6*(6), 318–323. https://doi.org/10.1089/chi.2010.0604.pers

Kirschenbaum, D. S., Craig, R. D., Kelly, K. P., & Germann, J. N. (2007). Treatment and innovation: Description and evaluation of new programs currently available for your patients. *Obesity Management, 3*(6), 261–266. https://doi.org/10.1089/obe.2007.0115

Klok, M. D., Jakobsdottir, S., & Drent, M. L. (2007). The role of leptin and ghrelin in the regulation of food intake and body weight in humans: A review. *Obesity Reviews, 8*(1), 21–34. https://doi.org/10.1111/j.1467-789X.2006.00270.x

Knowlden, A. P., & Conrad, E. (2018). Two-year outcomes of the Enabling Mothers to Prevent Pediatric Obesity through Web-Based Education and Reciprocal Determinism (EMPOWER) randomized control trial. *Health Education & Behavior, 45*(2), 262–276. https://doi.org/10.1177/1090198117732604

Knowlden, A., & Sharma, M. (2012). A feasibility and efficacy randomized controlled trial of an online preventative program for childhood obesity: Protocol for the EMPOWER intervention. *JMIR Research Protocols, 1*(1), e5. https://doi.org/10.2196/resprot.2141

Knowlden, A. P., Sharma, M., Cottrell, R. R., Wilson, B. R., & Johnson, M. L. (2015). Impact evaluation of Enabling Mothers to Prevent Pediatric Obesity through Web-Based Education and Reciprocal Determinism (EMPOWER) randomized control trial. *Health Education & Behavior, 42*(2), 171–184. https://doi.org/10.1177/1090198114547816

Kolko, D. J., Iselin, A. M., & Gully, K. J. (2011). Evaluation of the sustainability and clinical outcome of Alternatives for Families: A Cognitive–Behavioral Therapy (AF-CBT) in a child protection center. *Child Abuse & Neglect, 35*(2), 105–116. https://doi.org/10.1016/j.chiabu.2010.09.004

Kong, K. L., Anzman-Frasca, S., Burgess, B., Serwatka, C., White, H. I., & Holmbeck, K. (2023). Systematic review of general parenting intervention impacts on child weight as a secondary outcome. *Childhood Obesity*, *19*(5), 293–308. https://doi.org/10.1089/chi.2022.0056

Koyanagi, A., Veronese, N., Vancampfort, D., Stickley, A., Jackson, S. E., Oh, H., Shin, J. I., Haro, J. M., Stubbs, B., & Smith, L. (2020). Association of bullying victimization with overweight and obesity among adolescents from 41 low- and middle-income countries. *Pediatric Obesity*, *15*(1), e12571. https://doi.org/10.1111/ijpo.12571

Kravitz-Wirtz, N., Bruns, A., Aubel, A. J., Zhang, X., & Buggs, S. A. (2022). Inequities in community exposure to deadly gun violence by race/ethnicity, poverty, and neighborhood disadvantage among youth in large U.S. cities. *Journal of Urban Health*, *99*(4), 610–625. https://doi.org/10.1007/s11524-022-00656-0

Kremer, K. P., Flower, A., Huang, J., & Vaughn, M. G. (2016). Behavior problems and children's academic achievement: A test of growth-curve models with gender and racial differences. *Children and Youth Services Review*, *67*, 95–104. https://doi.org/10.1016/j.childyouth.2016.06.003

Kroenke, K., Spitzer, R. L., & Williams, J. B. (2001). The PHQ-9: Validity of a brief depression severity measure. *Journal of General Internal Medicine*, *16*(9), 606–613. https://doi.org/10.1046/j.1525-1497.2001.016009606.x

Kroenke, K., Spitzer, R. L., Williams, J. B., & Löwe, B. (2010). The Patient Health Questionnaire Somatic, Anxiety, and Depressive symptom scales: A systematic review. *General Hospital Psychiatry*, *32*(4), 345–359. https://doi.org/10.1016/j.genhosppsych.2010.03.006

Krukowski, R. A., West, D. S., Siddiqui, N. J., Bursac, Z., Phillips, M. M., & Raczynski, J. M. (2008). No change in weight-based teasing when school-based obesity policies are implemented. *Archives of Pediatrics & Adolescent Medicine*, *162*(10), 936–942. https://doi.org/10.1001/archpedi.162.10.936

Kuczmarski, R. J., Ogden, C. L., Grummer-Strawn, L. M., Flegal, K. M., Guo, S. S., Wei, R., Mei, Z., Curtin, L. R., Roche, A. F., & Johnson, C. L. (2000, June 8). *CDC growth charts: United States* (DHHS publication No. [PHS] 2000-1250). https://stacks.cdc.gov/view/cdc/11267

Kumanyika, S. K. (2008). Environmental influences on childhood obesity: Ethnic and cultural influences in context. *Physiology & Behavior*, *94*(1), 61–70. https://doi.org/10.1016/j.physbeh.2007.11.019

Kumanyika, S. K. (2019). A framework for increasing equity impact in obesity prevention. *American Journal of Public Health*, *109*(10), 1350–1357. https://doi.org/10.2105/AJPH.2019.305221

Kumanyika, S. K., Whitt-Glover, M. C., Gary, T. L., Prewitt, T. E., Odoms-Young, A. M., Banks-Wallace, J., Beech, B. M., Halbert, C. H., Karanja, N., Lancaster, K. J., & Samuel-Hodge, C. D. (2007). Expanding the obesity research paradigm to reach African American communities. *Preventing Chronic Disease*, *4*(4), A112.

Kumar, S., Croghan, I. T., Biggs, B. K., Croghan, K., Prissel, R., Fuehrer, D., Donelan-Dunlap, B., & Sood, A. (2018). Family-based mindful eating intervention in adolescents with obesity: A pilot randomized clinical trial. *Children (Basel)*, *5*(7), 93. https://doi.org/10.3390/children5070093

Kyle, T. K., Dhurandhar, E. J., & Allison, D. B. (2016). Regarding obesity as a disease: Evolving policies and their implications. *Endocrinology and Metabolism Clinics of North America*, *45*(3), 511–520. https://doi.org/10.1016/j.ecl.2016.04.004

Kyle, T. K., Stanford, F. C., & Nadglowski, J. F. (2018). Addressing weight stigma and opening doors for a patient-centered approach to childhood obesity. *Obesity*, *26*(3), 457–458. https://doi.org/10.1002/oby.22084

La Marra, M., Villano, I., Ilardi, C. R., Carosella, M., Staiano, M., Iavarone, A., Chieffi, S., Messina, G., Polito, R., Porro, C., Scarinci, A., Monda, V., Carotenuto, M., Di Maio, G., & Messina, A. (2022). Executive functions in overweight and obese treatment-seeking patients: Cross-sectional data and longitudinal perspectives. *Brain Sciences*, *12*(6), 777. https://doi.org/10.3390/brainsci12060777

Langer, S. L., Crain, A. L., Senso, M. M., Levy, R. L., & Sherwood, N. E. (2014). Predicting child physical activity and screen time: Parental support for physical activity and general parenting styles. *Journal of Pediatric Psychology*, *39*(6), 633–642. https://doi.org/10.1093/jpepsy/jsu021

La Puma, J. (2016). What is culinary medicine and what does it do? *Population Health Management*, *19*(1), 1–3. https://doi.org/10.1089/pop.2015.0003

Lassale, C., Batty, G. D., Baghdadli, A., Jacka, F., Sánchez-Villegas, A., Kivimäki, M., & Akbaraly, T. (2019). Healthy dietary indices and risk of depressive outcomes: A systematic review and meta-analysis of observational studies. *Molecular Psychiatry*, *24*(7), 965–986. https://doi.org/10.1038/s41380-018-0237-8

Laudenslager, M., Chaudhry, Z. W., Rajagopal, S., Clynes, S., & Gudzune, K. A. (2021). Commercial weight loss programs in the management of obesity: An update. *Current Obesity Reports*, *10*(2), 90–99. https://doi.org/10.1007/s13679-021-00428-y

Lavender, J. M., Wonderlich, S. A., Engel, S. G., Gordon, K. H., Kaye, W. H., & Mitchell, J. E. (2015). Dimensions of emotion dysregulation in anorexia nervosa and bulimia nervosa: A conceptual review of the empirical literature. *Clinical Psychology Review*, *40*, 111–122. https://doi.org/10.1016/j.cpr.2015.05.010

Lawlor, E. R., Islam, N., Bates, S., Griffin, S. J., Hill, A. J., Hughes, C. A., Sharp, S. J., & Ahern, A. L. (2020). Third-wave cognitive behaviour therapies for weight management: A systematic review and network meta-analysis. *Obesity Reviews*, *21*(7), e13013. https://doi.org/10.1111/obr.13013

Lawrence, S. E., Puhl, R. M., Schwartz, M. B., Watson, R. J., & Foster, G. D. (2022). "The most hurtful thing I've ever experienced": A qualitative examination of the nature of experiences of weight stigma by family members. *SSM—Qualitative Research in Health*, *2*, 100073. https://doi.org/10.1016/j.ssmqr.2022.100073

Learning Assistance Centre, University of Manitoba. (2023). *Goal setting*. https://umanitoba.ca/student/academiclearning/media/Goal-Setting-06.pdf

Lebow, J., Chuy, J. A., Cedermark, K., Cook, K., & Sim, L. A. (2015). The development or exacerbation of eating disorder symptoms after topiramate initiation. *Pediatrics*, *135*(5), e1312–e1316. https://doi.org/10.1542/peds.2014-3413

Lebow, J., Sim, L. A., & Kransdorf, L. N. (2015). Prevalence of a history of overweight and obesity in adolescents with restrictive eating disorders. *Journal of Adolescent Health, 56*(1), 19–24. https://doi.org/10.1016/j.jadohealth.2014.06.005

Lee, J. L., Eaton, C., Gutiérrez-Colina, A. M., Devine, K., Simons, L. E., Mee, L., & Blount, R. L. (2014). Longitudinal stability of specific barriers to medication adherence. *Journal of Pediatric Psychology, 39*(7), 667–676. https://doi.org/10.1093/jpepsy/jsu026

Lee, K. M., Arriola-Sanchez, L., Lumeng, J. C., Gearhardt, A., & Tomiyama, A. J. (2022). Weight stigma by association among parents of children with obesity: A randomized trial. *Academic Pediatrics, 22*(5), 754–760. https://doi.org/10.1016/j.acap.2021.09.019

Lee, S. H., Paz-Filho, G., Mastronardi, C., Licinio, J., & Wong, M.-L. (2016). Is increased antidepressant exposure a contributory factor to the obesity pandemic? *Translational Psychiatry, 6*(3), e759. https://doi.org/10.1038/tp.2016.25

Lee-Winn, A. E., Reinblatt, S. P., Mojtabai, R., & Mendelson, T. (2016). Gender and racial/ethnic differences in binge eating symptoms in a nationally representative sample of adolescents in the United States. *Eating Behaviors, 22,* 27–33. https://doi.org/10.1016/j.eatbeh.2016.03.021

Le Grange, D., Swanson, S. A., Crow, S. J., & Merikangas, K. R. (2012). Eating disorder not otherwise specified presentation in the US population. *International Journal of Eating Disorders, 45*(5), 711–718. https://doi.org/10.1002/eat.22006

Lessard, L. M., & Puhl, R. M. (2021). Reducing educators' weight Bias: The role of school-based anti-bullying policies. *Journal of School Health, 91*(10), 796–801. https://doi.org/10.1111/josh.13068

Lessard, L. M., Puhl, R. M., Larson, N., Simone, M., Eisenberg, M. E., & Neumark-Sztainer, D. (2021). Parental contributors to the prevalence and long-term health risks of family weight teasing in adolescence. *Journal of Adolescent Health, 69*(1), 74–81. https://doi.org/10.1016/j.jadohealth.2020.09.034

Leung, A. K. C., & Hon, K. L. (2019). Pica: A common condition that is commonly missed—An update review. *Current Pediatric Reviews, 15*(3), 164–169. https://doi.org/10.2174/1573396315666190313163530

Levi, J., Wang, J., Venter, F., & Hill, A. (2023). Estimated minimum prices and lowest available national prices for antiobesity medications: Improving affordability and access to treatment. *Obesity, 31*(5), 1270–1279. https://doi.org/10.1002/oby.23725

Levy, S. E., Pinto-Martin, J. A., Bradley, C. B., Chittams, J., Johnson, S. L., Pandey, J., Pomykacz, A., Ramirez, A., Reynolds, A., Rubenstein, E., Schieve, L. A., Shapira, S. K., Thompson, A., Young, L., & Kral, T. V. E. (2019). Relationship of weight outcomes, co-occurring conditions, and severity of autism spectrum disorder in the Study to Explore Early Development. *The Journal of Pediatrics, 205,* 202–209. https://doi.org/10.1016/j.jpeds.2018.09.003

Lim, C. S., Anderson, L. M., Hollingsworth, D. W., Shepherd, L., Sandridge, S., & Lanciers, S. (2019). Comparing disordered eating and feeding practices in

African American and Caucasian treatment-seeking youth with obesity. *Eating Disorders*, *27*(2), 152–167. https://doi.org/10.1080/10640266.2019.1614825

Lim, C. S., Espil, F. M., Viana, A. G., & Janicke, D. M. (2015). Associations between anxiety symptoms and child and family factors in pediatric obesity. *Journal of Developmental and Behavioral Pediatrics*, *36*(9), 664–672. https://doi.org/10.1097/DBP.0000000000000225

Lim, C. S., Gowey, M. A., & Janicke, D. M. (2014). Behavioral family treatment of pediatric obesity in an underserved community-based setting: A case study demonstrating barriers to treatment effectiveness. *Clinical Practice in Pediatric Psychology*, *2*(3), 236–249. https://doi.org/10.1037/cpp0000063

Lim, C. S., & Janicke, D. M. (2013). Barriers related to delivering pediatric weight management interventions to children and families from rural communities. *Children's Health Care*, *42*(3), 214–230. https://doi.org/10.1080/02739615.2013.816596

Lim, C. S., Robinson, J., Hinton, E., Gordy, X. Z., Gamble, A., Compretta, C., Holmes, M. E., & Ravola, M. (2022). School-based obesity prevention programs in rural communities: A scoping review. *JBI Evidence Synthesis*, *20*(12), 2936–2985. https://doi.org/10.11124/JBIES-21-00233

Lim, C. S., Schneider, E. M., & Janicke, D. M. (2018). Developmental influences on behavior change: Children, adolescents, emerging adults, and the elderly. In M. E. Hilliard, K. A. Riekert, J. K. Ockene, & L. Pbert (Eds.), *The handbook of health behavior change* (5th ed., pp. 75–101). Springer.

Lim, H. J., Xue, H., & Wang, Y. (2020). Global trends in obesity. In H. L. Meiselman (Ed.), *Handbook of eating and drinking: Interdisciplinary perspectives* (pp. 1217–1235). SpringerLink. https://doi.org/10.1007/978-3-030-14504-0_157

Limbers, C. A., Cohen, L. A., & Gray, B. A. (2018). Eating disorders in adolescent and young adult males: Prevalence, diagnosis, and treatment strategies. *Adolescent Health, Medicine and Therapeutics*, *9*, 111–116. https://doi.org/10.2147/AHMT.S147480

Lindberg, L., Hagman, E., Danielsson, P., Marcus, C., & Persson, M. (2020). Anxiety and depression in children and adolescents with obesity: A nationwide study in Sweden. *BMC Medicine*, *18*(1), 30. https://doi.org/10.1186/s12916-020-1498-z

Linehan, M. M. (1993a). *Cognitive–behavioral treatment of borderline personality disorder*. Guilford Press.

Linehan, M. M. (1993b). *Skills training manual for treating borderline personality disorder*. Guilford Press.

Ling, J., & Stommel, M. (2019). Parental and self-weight perceptions in U.S. children and adolescents, NHANES 2005–2014. *Western Journal of Nursing Research*, *41*(1), 42–57. https://doi.org/10.1177/0193945918758274

Lisse, A. A., Hochgraf, A. K., & McHale, S. M. (2022). Weight concerns in Black youth: The role of body mass index, gender, and sociocultural factors. *Journal of Research on Adolescence, 32*(4), 1341–1353. https://doi.org/10.1111/jora.12692

Locher, C., Koechlin, H., Zion, S. R., Werner, C., Pine, D. S., Kirsch, I., Kessler, R. C., & Kossowsky, J. (2017). Efficacy and safety of selective serotonin reuptake inhibitors, serotonin–norepinephrine reuptake inhibitors, and placebo for common psychiatric disorders among children and adolescents: A systematic review and meta-analysis. *JAMA Psychiatry, 74*(10), 1011–1020. https://doi.org/10.1001/jamapsychiatry.2017.2432

Lock, J. (2015). An update on evidence-based psychosocial treatments for eating disorders in children and adolescents. *Journal of Clinical Child & Adolescent Psychology, 44*(5), 707–721. https://doi.org/10.1080/15374416.2014.971458

Lock, J., & Le Grange, D. (2015). *Treatment manual for anorexia nervosa: A family-based approach.* Guilford Press.

Lumeng, J. C., Forrest, P., Appugliese, D. P., Kaciroti, N., Corwyn, R. F., & Bradley, R. H. (2010). Weight status as a predictor of being bullied in third through sixth grades. *Pediatrics, 125*(6), e1301–e1307. https://doi.org/10.1542/peds.2009-0774

Lumeng, J. C., Miller, A. L., Horodynski, M. A., Brophy-Herb, H. E., Contreras, D., Lee, H., Sturza, J., Kaciroti, N., & Peterson, K. E. (2017). Improving self-regulation for obesity prevention in Head Start: A randomized controlled trial. *Pediatrics, 139*(5), e20162047. https://doi.org/10.1542/peds.2016-2047

Luppino, F. S., de Wit, L. M., Bouvy, P. F., Stijnen, T., Cuijpers, P., Penninx, B. W., & Zitman, F. G. (2010). Overweight, obesity, and depression: A systematic review and meta-analysis of longitudinal studies. *Archives of General Psychiatry, 67*(3), 220–229. https://doi.org/10.1001/archgenpsychiatry.2010.2

Ma, L., Chu, M., Li, Y., Wu, Y., Yan, A. F., Johnson, B., & Wang, Y. (2021). Bidirectional relationships between weight stigma and pediatric obesity: A systematic review and meta-analysis. *Obesity Reviews, 22*(6), e13178. https://doi.org/10.1111/obr.13178

Mackey, E. R., Burton, E. T., Cadieux, A., Getzoff, E., Santos, M., Ward, W., & Beck, A. R. (2022). Addressing structural racism is critical for ameliorating the childhood obesity epidemic in Black youth. *Childhood Obesity, 18*(2), 75–83. https://doi.org/10.1089/chi.2021.0153

Mackey, E. R., Wang, J., Harrington, C., & Nadler, E. P. (2018). Psychiatric diagnoses and weight loss among adolescents receiving sleeve gastrectomy. *Pediatrics, 142*(1), e20173432. https://doi.org/10.1542/peds.2017-3432

Malacarne, D., Handakas, E., Robinson, O., Pineda, E., Saez, M., Chatzi, L., & Fecht, D. (2022). The built environment as determinant of childhood obesity: A systematic literature review. *Obesity Reviews, 23*(Suppl. 1), e13385. https://doi.org/10.1111/obr.13385

Maloney, M. J., McGuire, J. B., & Daniels, S. R. (1988). Reliability testing of a children's version of the Eating Attitude Test. *Journal of the American Academy of Child & Adolescent Psychiatry, 27*(5), 541–543. https://doi.org/10.1097/00004583-198809000-00004

Marcus, C., Danielsson, P., & Hagman, E. (2022). Pediatric obesity—Long-term consequences and effect of weight loss. *Journal of Internal Medicine, 292*(6), 870–891. https://doi.org/10.1111/joim.13547

Marques, L., Alegria, M., Becker, A. E., Chen, C. N., Fang, A., Chosak, A., & Diniz, J. B. (2011). Comparative prevalence, correlates of impairment, and service utilization for eating disorders across US ethnic groups: Implications for reducing ethnic disparities in health care access for eating disorders. *International Journal of Eating Disorders, 44*(5), 412–420. https://doi.org/10.1002/eat.20787

Marshall, H., & Albin, J. (2021). Food as medicine: A pilot nutrition and cooking curriculum for children of participants in a community-based culinary medicine class. *Maternal and Child Health Journal, 25*(1), 54–58. https://doi.org/10.1007/s10995-020-03031-0

Martins, R. K., & McNeil, D. W. (2009). Review of motivational interviewing in promoting health behaviors. *Clinical Psychology Review, 29*(4), 283–293. https://doi.org/10.1016/j.cpr.2009.02.001

Martinson, T. G., Ramachandran, S., Lindner, R., Reisman, T., & Safer, J. D. (2020). High body mass index is a significant barrier to gender-confirmation surgery for transgender and gender-nonbinary individuals. *Endocrine Practice, 26*(1), 6–15. https://doi.org/10.4158/EP-2019-0345

Masheb, R. M., & Grilo, C. M. (2006). Emotional overeating and its associations with eating disorder psychopathology among overweight patients with binge eating disorder. *International Journal of Eating Disorders, 39*(2), 141–146. https://doi.org/10.1002/eat.20221

Matheson, B. E., & Douglas, J. M. (2017). Overweight and obesity in children with autism spectrum disorder (ASD): A critical review investigating the etiology, development, and maintenance of this relationship. *Review Journal of Autism and Developmental Disorders, 4*(2), 142–156. https://doi.org/10.1007/s40489-017-0103-7

Matheson, B. E., & Eichen, D. M. (2018). A review of childhood behavioral problems and disorders in the development of obesity: Attention deficit/hyperactivity disorder, autism spectrum disorder, and beyond. *Current Obesity Reports, 7*(1), 19–26. https://doi.org/10.1007/s13679-018-0293-z

Matsui, D. (2007). Current issues in pediatric medication adherence. *Paediatric Drugs, 9*(5), 283–288. https://doi.org/10.2165/00148581-200709050-00001

McElroy, S. L., Hudson, J. I., Capece, J. A., Beyers, K., Fisher, A. C., Rosenthal, N. R., & the Topiramate Binge Eating Disorder Research Group. (2007). Topiramate for the treatment of binge eating disorder associated with obesity: A placebo-controlled study. *Biological Psychiatry, 61*(9), 1039–1048. https://doi.org/10.1016/j.biopsych.2006.08.008

McElroy, S. L., Hudson, J. I., Mitchell, J. E., Wilfley, D., Ferreira-Cornwell, M. C., Gao, J., Wang, J., Whitaker, T., Jonas, J., & Gasior, M. (2015). Efficacy and safety of lisdexamfetamine for treatment of adults with moderate to severe binge-eating disorder: A randomized clinical trial. *JAMA Psychiatry, 72*(3), 235–246. https://doi.org/10.1001/jamapsychiatry.2014.2162

McGrady, M. E., & Hommel, K. A. (2013). Medication adherence and health care utilization in pediatric chronic illness: A systematic review. *Pediatrics, 132*(4), 730–740. https://doi.org/10.1542/peds.2013-1451

Mechler, K., Banaschewski, T., Hohmann, S., & Hage, A. (2022). Evidence-based pharmacological treatment options for ADHD in children and adolescents. *Pharmacology & Therapeutics, 230*, 107940. https://doi.org/10.1016/j.pharmthera.2021.107940

Mensinger, J. L., Tylka, T. L., & Calamari, M. E. (2018). Mechanisms underlying weight status and healthcare avoidance in women: A study of weight stigma, body-related shame and guilt, and healthcare stress. *Body Image, 25*, 139–147. https://doi.org/10.1016/j.bodyim.2018.03.001

Mercado, D., Robinson, L., Gordon, G., Werthmann, J., Campbell, I. C., & Schmidt, U. (2021). The outcomes of mindfulness-based interventions for obesity and binge eating disorder: A meta-analysis of randomised controlled trials. *Appetite, 166*, 105464. https://doi.org/10.1016/j.appet.2021.105464

Merikangas, K. R., Nakamura, E. F., & Kessler, R. C. (2009). Epidemiology of mental disorders in children and adolescents. *Dialogues in Clinical Neuroscience, 11*(1), 7–20. https://doi.org/10.31887/DCNS.2009.11.1/krmerikangas

Merrill, B. M., Morrow, A. S., Sarver, D., Sandridge, S., & Lim, C. S. (2021). Prevalence and correlates of attention-deficit hyperactivity disorder in a diverse, treatment-seeking pediatric overweight/obesity sample. *Journal of Developmental & Behavioral Pediatrics, 42*(6), 433–441. https://doi.org/10.1097/DBP.0000000000000910

Messiah, S. E., Xie, L., Atem, F., Mathew, M. S., Qureshi, F. G., Schneider, B. E., & Cruz-Muñoz, N. (2022). Disparity between United States adolescent Class II and III obesity trends and bariatric surgery utilization, 2015–2018. *Annals of Surgery, 276*(2), 324–333. https://doi.org/10.1097/SLA.0000000000004493

Michaud, P.-A., Blum, R. W., Benaroyo, L., Zermatten, J., & Baltag, V. (2015). Assessing an adolescent's capacity for autonomous decision-making in clinical care. *Journal of Adolescent Health, 57*(4), 361–366. https://doi.org/10.1016/j.jadohealth.2015.06.012

Mikami, A. Y., Jia, M., & Na, J. J. (2014). Social skills training. *Child and Adolescent Psychiatric Clinics of North America, 23*(4), 775–788. https://doi.org/10.1016/j.chc.2014.05.007

Miller, A. L., Rathus, J. H., & Linehan, M. M. (2006). *Dialectical behavior therapy with suicidal adolescents*. Guilford Press.

Miller, J. L., & Tan, M. (2020). Dietary management for adolescents with Prader–Willi syndrome. *Adolescent Health, Medicine and Therapeutics, 11*, 113–118. https://doi.org/10.2147/AHMT.S214893

Min, J., Chiu, D. T., & Wang, Y. (2013). Variation in the heritability of body mass index based on diverse twin studies: A systematic review. *Obesity Reviews, 14*(11), 871–882. https://doi.org/10.1111/obr.12065

Minkovitz, C. S., Strobino, D., Mistry, K. B., Scharfstein, D. O., Grason, H., Hou, W., Ialongo, N., & Guyer, B. (2007). Healthy Steps for Young Children: Sustained results at 5.5 years. *Pediatrics, 120*(3), e658–e668. https://doi.org/10.1542/peds.2006-1205

Mitchell, J. A., Dowda, M., Pate, R. R., Kordas, K., Froberg, K., Sardinha, L. B., Kolle, E., & Page, A. (2017). Physical activity and pediatric obesity: A quantile regression analysis. *Medicine & Science in Sports & Exercise, 49*(3), 466–473. https://doi.org/10.1249/MSS.0000000000001129

Mitchell, J. E. (2016). Medical comorbidity and medical complications associated with binge-eating disorder. *International Journal of Eating Disorders, 49*(3), 319–323. https://doi.org/10.1002/eat.22452

Mitchison, D., Hay, P., Slewa-Younan, S., & Mond, J. (2014). The changing demographic profile of eating disorder behaviors in the community. *BMC Public Health, 14*(1), 943. https://doi.org/10.1186/1471-2458-14-943

Mitchison, D., Mond, J., Bussey, K., Griffiths, S., Trompeter, N., Lonergan, A., Pike, K. M., Murray, S. B., & Hay, P. (2020). *DSM-5* full syndrome, other specified, and unspecified eating disorders in Australian adolescents: Prevalence and clinical significance. *Psychological Medicine, 50*(6), 981–990. https://doi.org/10.1017/S0033291719000898

MO HealthNet Division, Missouri Department of Social Services. (2021). *Biopsychosocial treatment of obesity.* https://dss.mo.gov/mhd/providers/education/files/Biopsychosocial-Treatment-of-Obesity-09-21.pdf

Modi, A. C., Loux, T. J., Bell, S. K., Harmon, C. M., Inge, T. H., & Zeller, M. H. (2008). Weight-specific health-related quality of life in adolescents with extreme obesity. *Obesity, 16*(10), 2266–2271. https://doi.org/10.1038/oby.2008.347

Morrow, A. S., Sandridge, S., Herring, W., King, K., Lanciers, S., & Lim, C. S. (2020). Characterizing attendance patterns at a multidisciplinary pediatric obesity clinic. *Children's Health Care, 49*(3), 320–337. https://doi.org/10.1080/02739615.2020.1740884

Moskowitz, L., Lerman, J., DeVoe, C., & Attia, E. (2014). The eating disorders diagnoses: What has changed with *DSM-5.* In I. Dancyger & V. Fornari (Eds.), *Evidence based treatments for eating disorders: Children, adolescents, and adults* (pp. 105–126). Nova Science.

Moskowitz, L., & Weiselberg, E. (2017). Anorexia nervosa/atypical anorexia nervosa. *Current Problems in Pediatric and Adolescent Health Care, 47*(4), 70–84. https://doi.org/10.1016/j.cppeds.2017.02.003

Motevalli, M., Drenowatz, C., Tanous, D. R., Khan, N. A., & Wirnitzer, K. (2021). Management of childhood obesity—Time to shift from generalized to personalized intervention strategies. *Nutrients, 13*(4), 1200. https://doi.org/10.3390/nu13041200

Mühlig, Y., Antel, J., Föcker, M., & Hebebrand, J. (2016). Are bidirectional associations of obesity and depression already apparent in childhood and adolescence as based on high-quality studies? A systematic review. *Obesity Reviews, 17*(3), 235–249. https://doi.org/10.1111/obr.12357

Murphy, J. M., Bergmann, P., Chiang, C., Sturner, R., Howard, B., Abel, M. R., & Jellinek, M. (2016). The PSC-17: Subscale scores, reliability, and factor structure in a new national sample. *Pediatrics, 138*(3), e20160038. https://doi.org/10.1542/peds.2016-0038

Nam, H. K., & Lee, K. H. (2018). Small for gestational age and obesity: Epidemiology and general risks. *Annals of Pediatric Endocrinology & Metabolism, 23*(1), 9–13. https://doi.org/10.6065/apem.2018.23.1.9

National Heart, Lung, and Blood Institute. (2018). *Healthy Communities Study (HCS)*. https://biolincc.nhlbi.nih.gov/studies/hcs/

National Institute of Mental Health. (2016). *Eating disorders—Binge eating disorder*. https://www.nimh.nih.gov/health/statistics/prevalence/eating-disorders-among-adults-binge-eating-disorder.shtml

Neblett, E. W., Jr. (2019). Racism and health: Challenges and future directions in behavioral and psychological research. *Cultural Diversity and Ethnic Minority Psychology, 25*(1), 12–20. https://doi.org/10.1037/cdp0000253

Neumark-Sztainer, D. (2009). Preventing obesity and eating disorders in adolescents: What can health care providers do? *Journal of Adolescent Health, 44*(3), 206–213. https://doi.org/10.1016/j.jadohealth.2008.11.005

Neumark-Sztainer, D., Falkner, N., Story, M., Perry, C., Hannan, P. J., & Mulert, S. (2002). Weight-teasing among adolescents: Correlations with weight status and disordered eating behaviors. *International Journal of Obesity, 26*(1), 123–131. https://doi.org/10.1038/sj.ijo.0801853

Nguyen, C. T., Fairclough, D. L., & Noll, R. B. (2016). Problem-solving skills training for mothers of children recently diagnosed with autism spectrum disorder: A pilot feasibility study. *Autism, 20*(1), 55–64. https://doi.org/10.1177/1362361314567134

Nujić, D., Musić Milanović, S., Milas, V., Miškulin, I., Ivić, V., & Milas, J. (2021). Association between child/adolescent overweight/obesity and conduct disorder: A systematic review and meta-analysis. *Pediatric Obesity, 16*(5), e12742. https://doi.org/10.1111/ijpo.12742

Nuttall, F. Q. (2015). Body mass index: Obesity, BMI, and health: A critical review. *Nutrition Today, 50*(3), 117–128. https://doi.org/10.1097/NT.0000000000000092

Nutter, S., Ireland, A., Alberga, A. S., Brun, I., Lefebvre, D., Hayden, K. A., & Russell-Mayhew, S. (2019). Weight bias in educational settings: A systematic review. *Current Obesity Reports, 8*(2), 185–200. https://doi.org/10.1007/s13679-019-00330-8

Obesity Action Coalition. (2022). *People-first language*. https://www.obesityaction.org/advocacy/what-we-fight-for/people-first-language

The Obesity Society. (2015). *Potential contributors to obesity*. https://www.obesity.org/wp-content/uploads/2020/05/TOS-Reasons-for-obesity-infographic-2015.pdf

Ogden, C. L., Carroll, M. D., Fakhouri, T. H., Hales, C. M., Fryar, C. D., Li, X., & Freedman, D. S. (2018). Prevalence of obesity among youths by household income and education level of head of household—United States 2011–2014.

Morbidity and Mortality Weekly Report, 67(6), 186–189. https://doi.org/10.15585/mmwr.mm6706a3

Ogden, C. L., Fryar, C. D., Martin, C. B., Freedman, D. S., Carroll, M. D., Gu, Q., & Hales, C. M. (2020). Trends in obesity prevalence by race and Hispanic origin—1999–2000 to 2017–2018. *JAMA, 324*(12), 1208–1210. https://doi.org/10.1001/jama.2020.14590

Ohri-Vachaspati, P., Acciai, F., Lloyd, K., Tulloch, D., DeWeese, R. S., DeLia, D., Todd, M., & Yedidia, M. J. (2021). Evidence that changes in community food environments lead to changes in children's weight: Results from a longitudinal prospective cohort study. *Journal of the Academy of Nutrition and Dietetics, 121*(3), 419–434. https://doi.org/10.1016/j.jand.2020.10.016

Osuchukwu, O. O., & Reed, D. J. (2022). Small for gestational age. *StatPearls.* https://www.ncbi.nlm.nih.gov/books/NBK563247/

Pai, A. L., & McGrady, M. (2014). Systematic review and meta-analysis of psychological interventions to promote treatment adherence in children, adolescents, and young adults with chronic illness. *Journal of Pediatric Psychology, 39*(8), 918–931. https://doi.org/10.1093/jpepsy/jsu038

Palad, C. J., Yarlagadda, S., & Stanford, F. C. (2019). Weight stigma and its impact on paediatric care. *Current Opinion in Endocrinology, Diabetes, and Obesity, 26*(1), 19–24. https://doi.org/10.1097/MED.0000000000000453

Palermo, T. M., Law, E. F., Essner, B., Jessen-Fiddick, T., & Eccleston, C. (2014). Adaptation of Problem-Solving Skills Training (PSST) for parent caregivers of youth with chronic Pain. *Clinical Practice in Pediatric Psychology, 2*(3), 212–223. https://doi.org/10.1037/cpp0000067

Pate, R. R., Frongillo, E. A., McIver, K. L., Colabianchi, N., Wilson, D. K., Collie-Akers, V. L., Schultz, J. A., Reis, J., Madsen, K., Woodward-Lopez, G., Berrigan, D., Landgraf, A., Nagaraja, J., Strauss, W. J., & the Healthy Communities Study Team. (2018). Associations between community programmes and policies and children's physical activity: The Healthy Communities Study. *Pediatric Obesity, 13*(Suppl. 1), 72–81. https://doi.org/10.1111/ijpo.12426

Patel, A. I., Madsen, K. A., Maselli, J. H., Cabana, M. D., Stafford, R. S., & Hersh, A. L. (2010). Underdiagnosis of pediatric obesity during outpatient preventive care visits. *Academic Pediatrics, 10*(6), 405–409. https://doi.org/10.1016/j.acap.2010.09.004

Patrick, D. L., Skalicky, A. M., Edwards, T. C., Kuniyuki, A., Morales, L. S., Leng, M., & Kirschenbaum, D. S. (2011). Weight loss and changes in generic and weight-specific quality of life in obese adolescents. *Quality of Life Research, 20*(6), 961–968. https://doi.org/10.1007/s11136-010-9824-0

Pearl, R. L., Allison, K. C., Shaw Tronieri, J., & Wadden, T. A. (2018). Reconsidering the psychosocial–behavioral evaluation required prior to bariatric surgery. *Obesity, 26*(2), 249–250. https://doi.org/10.1002/oby.22063

Pearl, R. L., Dovidio, J. F., & Puhl, R. M. (2015). Visual portrayals of obesity in health media: Promoting exercise without perpetuating weight bias. *Health Education Research, 30*(4), 580–590. https://doi.org/10.1093/her/cyv025

Pearl, R. L., Puhl, R. M., & Brownell, K. D. (2012). Positive media portrayals of obese persons: Impact on attitudes and image preferences. *Health Psychology, 31*(6), 821–829. https://doi.org/10.1037/a0027189

Perez, N. P., Westfal, M. L., Stapleton, S. M., Stanford, F. C., Griggs, C. L., Pratt, J. S., Chang, D. C., & Kelleher, C. M. (2020). Beyond insurance: Race-based disparities in the use of metabolic and bariatric surgery for the management of severe pediatric obesity. *Surgery for Obesity and Related Diseases, 16*(3), 414–419. https://doi.org/10.1016/j.soard.2019.11.020

Pervanidou, P., & Chrousos, G. P. (2011). Stress and obesity/metabolic syndrome in childhood and adolescence. *International Journal of Pediatric Obesity, 6*(Suppl. 1), 21–28. https://doi.org/10.3109/17477166.2011.615996

Peterson, C. M., Van Diest, A. M. K., Mara, C. A., & Matthews, A. (2020). Dialectical behavioral therapy skills group as an adjunct to family-based therapy in adolescents with restrictive eating disorders. *Eating Disorders, 28*(1), 67–79. https://doi.org/10.1080/10640266.2019.1568101

Phillips, B. A., Gaudette, S., McCracken, A., Razzaq, S., Sutton, K., Speed, L., Thompson, J., & Ward, W. (2012). Psychosocial functioning in children and adolescents with extreme obesity. *Journal of Clinical Psychology in Medical Settings, 19*(3), 277–284. https://doi.org/10.1007/s10880-011-9293-9

Pidano, A. E., & Allen, A. R. (2015). The Incredible Years series: A review of the independent research base. *Journal of Child and Family Studies, 24*(7), 1898–1916. https://doi.org/10.1007/s10826-014-9991-7

Pirgon, Ö., & Aslan, N. (2015). The role of urbanization in childhood obesity. *Journal of Clinical Research in Pediatric Endocrinology, 7*(3), 163–167. https://doi.org/10.4274/jcrpe.1984

Plevinsky, J. M., Gutierrez-Colina, A. M., Carmody, J. K., Hommel, K. A., Crosby, L. E., McGrady, M. E., Pai, A. L. H., Ramsey, R. R., & Modi, A. C. (2020). Patient-reported outcomes for pediatric adherence and self-management: A systematic review. *Journal of Pediatric Psychology, 45*(3), 340–357. https://doi.org/10.1093/jpepsy/jsz096

Plevinsky, J. M., Young, M. A., Carmody, J. K., Durkin, L. K., Gamwell, K. L., Klages, K. L., Ghosh, S., & Hommel, K. A. (2020). The impact of COVID-19 on pediatric adherence and self-management. *Journal of Pediatric Psychology, 45*(9), 977–982. https://doi.org/10.1093/jpepsy/jsaa079

Pluhar, E. I., Kamody, R. C., Sanchez, J., Thurston, I. B., & Burton, E. T. (2018). Description of an intervention to treat binge-eating behaviors among adolescents: Applying the Template for Intervention Descriptions and Replication. *International Journal of Eating Disorders, 51*(10), 1128–1133. https://doi.org/10.1002/eat.22954

Pomeroy, J., Krentz, A. D., Richardson, J. G., Berg, R. L., VanWormer, J. J., & Haws, R. M. (2021). Bardet–Biedl syndrome: Weight patterns and genetics in a rare obesity syndrome. *Pediatric Obesity, 16*(2), e12703. https://doi.org/10.1111/ijpo.12703

Pont, S. J., Puhl, R., Cook, S. R., Slusser, W., Section on Obesity, & the Obesity Society. (2017). Stigma experienced by children and adolescents with obesity. *Pediatrics, 140*(6), e20173034. https://doi.org/10.1542/peds.2017-3034

Pratt, J. S. A., Browne, A., Browne, N. T., Bruzoni, M., Cohen, M., Desai, A., Inge, T., Linden, B. C., Mattar, S. G., Michalsky, M., Podkameni, D., Reichard, K. W., Stanford, F. C., Zeller, M. H., & Zitsman, J. (2018). ASMBS pediatric metabolic and bariatric surgery guidelines, 2018. *Surgery for Obesity and Related Diseases, 14*(7), 882–901. https://doi.org/10.1016/j.soard.2018.03.019

Pratt, L. A., Brody, D. J., & Gu, Q. (2017, August). *Antidepressant use among persons aged 12 and over: United States, 2011–2014*. NCHS Data Brief No. 283. https://www.cdc.gov/nchs/products/databriefs/db283.htm#:~:text=During%202011%E2%80%932014%2C%2012.7%25,race%20and%20Hispanic%2Dorigin%20groups

Pugliese, J., & Tinsley, B. (2007). Parental socialization of child and adolescent physical activity: A meta-analysis. *Journal of Family Psychology, 21*(3), 331–343. https://doi.org/10.1037/0893-3200.21.3.331

Puhl, R. (2013). Obesity stigma: Implications for patients and providers [PowerPoint Slides]. Rudd Center for Food Policy & Obesity, Yale University.

Puhl, R. M., Andreyeva, T., & Brownell, K. D. (2008). Perceptions of weight discrimination: Prevalence and comparison to race and gender discrimination in America. *International Journal of Obesity, 32*(6), 992–1000. https://doi.org/10.1038/ijo.2008.22

Puhl, R. M., & Heuer, C. A. (2009). The stigma of obesity: A review and update. *Obesity, 17*(5), 941–964. https://doi.org/10.1038/oby.2008.636

Puhl, R. M., & Heuer, C. A. (2010). Obesity stigma: Important considerations for public health. *American Journal of Public Health, 100*(6), 1019–1028. https://doi.org/10.2105/AJPH.2009.159491

Puhl, R. M., Himmelstein, M. S., & Pearl, R. L. (2020). Weight stigma as a psychosocial contributor to obesity. *American Psychologist, 75*(2), 274–289. https://doi.org/10.1037/amp0000538

Puhl, R. M., Himmelstein, M. S., & Quinn, D. M. (2018). Internalizing weight stigma: Prevalence and sociodemographic considerations in US adults. *Obesity, 26*(1), 167–175. https://doi.org/10.1002/oby.22029

Puhl, R. M., & King, K. M. (2013). Weight discrimination and bullying. *Best Practice & Research: Clinical Endocrinology & Metabolism, 27*(2), 117–127. https://doi.org/10.1016/j.beem.2012.12.002

Puhl, R. M., & Latner, J. D. (2007). Stigma, obesity, and the health of the nation's children. *Psychological Bulletin, 133*(4), 557–580. https://doi.org/10.1037/0033-2909.133.4.557

Puhl, R. M., Latner, J. D., King, K. M., & Luedicke, J. (2014). Weight bias among professionals treating eating disorders: Attitudes about treatment and perceived patient outcomes. *International Journal of Eating Disorders, 47*(1), 65–75. https://doi.org/10.1002/eat.22186

Puhl, R. M., & Lessard, L. M. (2020). Weight stigma in youth: Prevalence, consequences, and considerations for clinical practice. *Current Obesity Reports, 9*(4), 402–411. https://doi.org/10.1007/s13679-020-00408-8

Puhl, R. M., & Luedicke, J. (2012). Weight-based victimization among adolescents in the school setting: Emotional reactions and coping behaviors. *Journal of Youth and Adolescence, 41*(1), 27–40. https://doi.org/10.1007/s10964-011-9713-z

Puhl, R. M., Moss-Racusin, C. A., Schwartz, M. B., & Brownell, K. D. (2008). Weight stigmatization and bias reduction: Perspectives of overweight and obese adults. *Health Education Research, 23*(2), 347–358. https://doi.org/10.1093/her/cym052

Puhl, R. M., Peterson, J. L., & Luedicke, J. (2013). Weight-based victimization: Bullying experiences of weight loss treatment-seeking youth. *Pediatrics, 131*(1), e1–e9. https://doi.org/10.1542/peds.2012-1106

Puhl, R. M., & Suh, Y. (n.d.). *Weight bias in clinical care: Improving health care for patients with overweight and obesity*. https://uconnruddcenter.org/wp-content/uploads/sites/2909/2020/07/CME-Complete-with-links.pdf

Puhl, R. M., Wall, M. M., Chen, C., Bryn Austin, S., Eisenberg, M. E., & Neumark-Sztainer, D. (2017). Experiences of weight teasing in adolescence and weight-related outcomes in adulthood: A 15-year longitudinal study. *Preventive Medicine, 100*, 173–179. https://doi.org/10.1016/j.ypmed.2017.04.023

Puig, E. P., Robles, N., Saigí-Rubió, F., Zamora, A., Moharra, M., Paluzie, G., Balfegó, M., Cambra, G. C., Garcia-Lorda, P., & Carrion, C. (2019). Assessment of the efficacy, safety, and effectiveness of weight control and obesity management mobile health interventions: Systematic review. *JMIR mHealth and uHealth, 7*(10), e12612. https://doi.org/10.2196/12612

Pulgarón, E. R. (2013). Childhood obesity: A review of increased risk for physical and psychological comorbidities. *Clinical Therapeutics, 35*(1), A18–A32. https://doi.org/10.1016/j.clinthera.2012.12.014

Putnick, D. L., Bell, E. M., Ghassabian, A., Robinson, S. L., Sundaram, R., & Yeung, E. (2022). Feeding problems as an indicator of developmental delay in early childhood. *Journal of Pediatrics, 242*, P184–P191.E5. https://doi.org/10.1016/j.jpeds.2021.11.010

Quittner, A. L., Drotar, D., Ievers-Landis, C., Slocum, N., Seidner, D., & Jacobsen, J. (2000). Adherence to medical treatments in adolescents with cystic fibrosis: The development and evaluation of family-based interventions. In D. Drotar (Ed.), *Promoting adherence to medical treatments in chronic childhood illness* (pp. 383–407). Erlbaum.

Rahman, M., & Berenson, A. B. (2010). Accuracy of current body mass index obesity classification for White, Black, and Hispanic reproductive-age women. *Obstetrics and Gynecology, 115*(5), 982–988. https://doi.org/10.1097/AOG.0b013e3181da9423

Rankin, J., Matthews, L., Cobley, S., Han, A., Sanders, R., Wiltshire, H. D., & Baker, J. S. (2016). Psychological consequences of childhood obesity: Psychiatric comorbidity and prevention. *Adolescent Health, Medicine and Therapeutics, 7*, 125–146. https://doi.org/10.2147/AHMT.S101631

Rapoff, M. A., & Rapoff, M. A. (2010). Consequences of nonadherence and correlates of adherence. In *Adherence to pediatric medical regimens* (2nd ed., pp. 33–45). Springer. https://doi.org/10.1007/978-1-4419-0570-3_2

Rathbone, J. A., Cruwys, T., Jetten, J., & Barlow, F. K. (2023). When stigma is the norm: How weight and social norms influence the healthcare we receive. *Journal of Applied Social Psychology, 53*(3), 185–201. https://doi.org/10.1111/jasp.12689

Rathus, J. H., & Miller, A. L. (2014). *DBT skills manual for adolescents*. Guilford Press.

Reekie, J., Hosking, S. P. M., Prakash, C., Kao, K. T., Juonala, M., & Sabin, M. A. (2015). The effect of antidepressants and antipsychotics on weight gain in children and adolescents. *Obesity Reviews, 16*(7), 566–580. https://doi.org/10.1111/obr.12284

Reeves, G. M., Postolache, T. T., & Snitker, S. (2008). Childhood obesity and depression: Connection between these growing problems in growing children. *International Journal of Child Health and Human Development, 1*(2), 103–114.

Reilly, E. E., Orloff, N. C., Luo, T., Berner, L. A., Brown, T. A., Claudat, K., Kaye, W. H., & Anderson, L. K. (2020). Dialectical behavioral therapy for the treatment of adolescent eating disorders: A review of existing work and proposed future directions. *Eating Disorders, 28*(2), 122–141. https://doi.org/10.1080/10640266.2020.1743098

Reisig, V., & Wildner, M. (2008). Prevention, primary. In W. Kirch (Ed.), *Encyclopedia of public health* (pp. 1141–1143). Springer. https://doi.org/10.1007/978-1-4020-5614-7_2759

Resnicow, K., Davis, R., & Rollnick, S. (2006). Motivational interviewing for pediatric obesity: Conceptual issues and evidence review. *Journal of the American Dietetic Association, 106*(12), 2024–2033. https://doi.org/10.1016/j.jada.2006.09.015

Reynolds, C. R., & Kamphaus, R. W. (2015). *Behavior assessment system for children* (3rd ed.). Pearson.

Rhee, K. E., Lumeng, J. C., Appugliese, D. P., Kaciroti, N., & Bradley, R. H. (2006). Parenting styles and overweight status in first grade. *Pediatrics, 117*(6), 2047–2054. https://doi.org/10.1542/peds.2005-2259

Rhythm Pharmaceuticals. (2021). *Uncovering rare obesity*. https://uncoveringrareobesity.com/

Ricks, T. N., Abbyad, C., & Polinard, E. (2022). Undoing racism and mitigating bias among healthcare professionals: Lessons learned during a systematic review. *Journal of Racial and Ethnic Health Disparities, 9*(5), 1990–2000. https://doi.org/10.1007/s40615-021-01137-x

Riise, E. N., Wergeland, G. J. H., Njardvik, U., & Ost, L. G. (2021). Cognitive behavior therapy for externalizing disorders in children and adolescents in routine clinical care: A systematic review and meta-analysis. *Clinical Psychology Review, 83*, 101954. https://doi.org/10.1016/j.cpr.2020.101954

Rincon-Subtirelu, M. (2017). Education as a tool to modify anti-obesity bias among pediatric residents. *International Journal of Medical Education, 8*, 77–78. https://doi.org/10.5116/ijme.58b1.46e3

Ritchie, L. D., Woodward-Lopez, G., Au, L. E., Loria, C. M., Collie-Akers, V., Wilson, D. K., Frongillo, E. A., Strauss, W. J., Landgraf, A. J., Nagaraja, J., Sagatov, R. D. F., Nicastro, H. L., Nebeling, L. C., Webb, K. L., & the Health Communities Study Team. (2018). Associations of community programs and policies with children's dietary intakes: The Healthy Communities Study. *Pediatric Obesity, 13*(Suppl. 1), 14–26. https://doi.org/10.1111/ijpo.12440

Robinson, J. C., Lim, C. S., Hinton, E., Pintado, I., Gamble, A., Compretta, C., & Ravola, M. (2019). School-based obesity prevention programs in rural communities: A scoping review protocol. *JBI Database of Systematic Reviews and Implementation Reports, 17*(7), 1326–1333. https://doi.org/10.11124/JBISRIR-2017-003957

Rogers, J. M., Ferrari, M., Mosely, K., Lang, C. P., & Brennan, L. (2017). Mindfulness-based interventions for adults who are overweight or obese: A meta-analysis of physical and psychological health outcomes. *Obesity Reviews, 18*(1), 51–67. https://doi.org/10.1111/obr.12461

Rollnick, S., Miller, W. R., & Butler, C. C. (2008). *Motivational Interviewing in health care: Helping patients change behavior*. Guilford Press.

Rosen, D. S., & the Committee on Adolescence. (2010). Identification and management of eating disorders in children and adolescents. *Pediatrics, 126*(6), 1240–1253. https://doi.org/10.1542/peds.2010-2821

Rosenstock, J., Frias, J., Jastreboff, A. M., Du, Y., Lou, J., Gurbuz, S., Thomas, M. K., Hartman, M. L., Haupt, A., Milicevic, Z., & Coskun, T. (2023). Retatrutide, a GIP, GLP-1 and glucagon receptor agonist, for people with type 2 diabetes: A randomised, double-blind, placebo and active-controlled, parallel-group, Phase 2 trial conducted in the USA. *The Lancet, 402*(10401), 529–544. https://doi.org/10.1016/S0140-6736(23)01053-X

Ross, M. M., Kolbash, S., Cohen, G. M., & Skelton, J. A. (2010). Multidisciplinary treatment of pediatric obesity: Nutrition evaluation and management. *Nutrition in Clinical Practice, 25*(4), 327–334. https://doi.org/10.1177/0884533610373771

Rubino, F., Puhl, R. M., Cummings, D. E., Eckel, R. H., Ryan, D. H., Mechanick, J. I., Nadglowski, J., Ramos Salas, X., Schauer, P. R., Twenefour, D., Apovian, C. M., Aronne, L. J., Batterham, R. L., Berthoud, H. R., Boza, C., Busetto, L., Dicker, D., De Groot, M., Eisenberg, D., . . . Dixon, J. B. (2020). Joint international consensus statement for ending stigma of obesity. *Nature Medicine, 26*(4), 485–497. https://doi.org/10.1038/s41591-020-0803-x

Ruffman, T., O'Brien, K. S., Taumoepeau, M., Latner, J. D., & Hunter, J. A. (2016). Toddlers' bias to look at average versus obese figures relates to maternal anti-fat prejudice. *Journal of Experimental Child Psychology, 142*, 195–202. https://doi.org/10.1016/j.jecp.2015.10.008

Ryan, D. H., & Yockey, S. R. (2017). Weight loss and improvement in comorbidity: Differences at 5%, 10%, 15%, and over. *Current Obesity Reports, 6*(2), 187–194. https://doi.org/10.1007/s13679-017-0262-y

Ryder, J. R., Kaizer, A., Rudser, K. D., Gross, A., Kelly, A. S., & Fox, C. K. (2017). Effect of phentermine on weight reduction in a pediatric weight management clinic. *International Journal of Obesity, 41*(1), 90–93. https://doi.org/10.1038/ijo.2016.185

Sabin, J. A., Marini, M., & Nosek, B. A. (2012). Implicit and explicit anti-fat bias among a large sample of medical doctors by BMI, race/ethnicity and gender. *PLOS One, 7*(11), e48448. https://doi.org/10.1371/journal.pone.0048448

Sackey, J., DallaPiazza, M., Bentsianov, S., & Finkel, D. (2021). Overweight and obesity among adults identifying on the transgender spectrum in Newark, NJ between 2018 and 2020: A retrospective chart review. *Current Developments in Nutrition, 5,* 1244. https://doi.org/10.1093/cdn/nzab055_054

Safer, D. L., & Jo, B. (2010). Outcome from a randomized controlled trial of group therapy for binge eating disorder: Comparing dialectical behavior therapy adapted for binge eating to an active comparison group therapy. *Behavior Therapy, 41*(1), 106–120. https://doi.org/10.1016/j.beth.2009.01.006

Safer, D. L., Telch, C. F., & Chen, E. Y. (2009). *Dialectical behavior therapy for binge eating and bulimia.* Guilford Press.

Sagar, R., & Gupta, T. (2018). Psychological aspects of obesity in children and adolescents. *Indian Journal of Pediatrics, 85*(7), 554–559. https://doi.org/10.1007/s12098-017-2539-2

Sahler, O. J., Dolgin, M. J., Phipps, S., Fairclough, D. L., Askins, M. A., Katz, E. R., Noll, R. B., & Butler, R. W. (2013). Specificity of problem-solving skills training in mothers of children newly diagnosed with cancer: Results of a multisite randomized clinical trial. *Journal of Clinical Oncology, 31*(10), 1329–1335. https://doi.org/10.1200/JCO.2011.39.1870

St. Pierre, C., Ver Ploeg, M., Dietz, W. H., Pryor, S., Jakazi, C. S., Layman, E., Noymer, D., Coughtrey-Davenport, T., & Sacheck, J. M. (2022). Food insecurity and childhood obesity: A systematic review. *Pediatrics, 150*(1), 1–15. https://doi.org/10.1542/peds.2021-055571

Sammels, O., Karjalainen, L., Dahlgren, J., & Wentz, E. (2022). Autism spectrum disorder and obesity in children: A systematic review and meta-analysis. *Obesity Facts, 15*(3), 305–320. https://doi.org/10.1159/000523943

Sánchez-SanSegundo, M., Zaragoza-Martí, A., Martin-LLaguno, I., Berbegal, M., Ferrer-Cascales, R., & Hurtado-Sánchez, J. A. (2021). The role of BMI, body fat mass and visceral fat in executive function in individuals with overweight and obesity. *Nutrients, 13*(7), 2259. https://doi.org/10.3390/nu13072259

Sanders, L. M., Perrin, E. M., Yin, H. S., Delamater, A. M., Flower, K. B., Bian, A. H., Schildcrout, J. S., Rothman, R. L., & Greenlight Study Team. (2021). A health-literacy intervention for early childhood obesity prevention: A cluster-randomized controlled trial. *Pediatrics, 147*(5), e202004986. https://doi.org/10.1542/peds.2020-049866

Santos, M., Burton, E. T., Cadieux, A., Gaffka, B., Shaffer, L., Cook, J. L., & Tucker, J. M. (2022). Adverse childhood experiences, health behaviors, and associations with obesity among youth in the United States. *Behavioral Medicine.* Advance online publication. https://doi.org/10.1080/08964289.2022.2077294

Sarno, L. A., Lipshultz, S. E., Harmon, C., De La Cruz-Munoz, N. F., & Balakrishnan, P. L. (2020). Short- and long-term safety and efficacy of bariatric surgery for severely obese adolescents: A narrative review. *Pediatric Research, 87*(2), 202–209. https://doi.org/10.1038/s41390-019-0532-3

Sawyer, S. M., Whitelaw, M., Le Grange, D., Yeo, M., & Hughes, E. K. (2016). Physical and psychological morbidity in adolescents with atypical anorexia nervosa. *Pediatrics, 137*(4), e20154080. https://doi.org/10.1542/peds.2015-4080

Scheen, A. J. (2011). Sibutramine on cardiovascular outcome. *Diabetes Care, 34*(Suppl. 2), S114–S119. https://doi.org/10.2337/dc11-s205

Schlaudecker, E. P., Munoz, F. M., Bardají, A., Boghossian, N. S., Khalil, A., Mousa, H., Nesin, M., Nisar, M. I., Pool, V., Spiegel, H. M. L., Tapia, M. D., Kochhar, S., Black, S., & Brighton Collaboration Small for Gestational Age Working Group. (2017). Small for gestational age: Case definition and guidelines for data collection, analysis, and presentation of maternal immunisation safety data. *Vaccine, 35*(48, Pt. A), 6518–6528. https://doi.org/10.1016/j.vaccine.2017.01.040

Schoffman, D. E., Turner-McGrievy, G., Jones, S. J., & Wilcox, S. (2013). Mobile apps for pediatric obesity prevention and treatment, healthy eating, and physical activity promotion: Just fun and games? *Translational Behavioral Medicine, 3*(3), 320–325. https://doi.org/10.1007/s13142-013-0206-3

Schrempft, S., van Jaarsveld, C. H. M., Fisher, A., Herle, M., Smith, A. D., Fildes, A., & Llewellyn, C. H. (2018). Variation in the Heritability of Child Body Mass Index by obesogenic home environment. *JAMA Pediatrics, 172*(12), 1153–1160. https://doi.org/10.1001/jamapediatrics.2018.1508

Schroeder, K., Schuler, B. R., Kobulsky, J. M., & Sarwer, D. B. (2021). The association between adverse childhood experiences and childhood obesity: A systematic review. *Obesity Reviews, 22*(7), e13204. https://doi.org/10.1111/obr.13204

Schwimmer, J. B., Burwinkle, T. M., & Varni, J. W. (2003). Health-related quality of life of severely obese children and adolescents. *JAMA, 289*(14), 1813–1819. https://doi.org/10.1001/jama.289.14.1813

Section on Breastfeeding, Eidelman, A. I., Schanler, R. J., Johnston, M., Landers, S., Noble, L., . . . & Viehmann, L. (2012). Breastfeeding and the use of human milk. *Pediatrics, 129*(3), e827–e841. https://doi.org/10.1542/peds.2011-3552

Seid, M., Varni, J. W., Gidwani, P., Gelhard, L. R., & Slymen, D. J. (2010). Problem-solving skills training for vulnerable families of children with persistent asthma: Report of a randomized trial on health-related quality of life outcomes. *Journal of Pediatric Psychology, 35*(10), 1133–1143. https://doi.org/10.1093/jpepsy/jsp133

The $72 billion weight loss and diet control market in the United States, 2019–2023: Why meal replacements are still booming, but not OTC diet pills. (2019, February 25). Associated Press. https://apnews.com/press-release/business-wire/business-lifestyle-health-united-states-ec35f-3315f9a4816985615391f41815a

Shepherd, L. M., Sandridge, S., King, K., Herring, W., Lanciers, S., & Lim, C. S. (2018, November 11–15). *Physical activity and dietary behaviors in children with obesity and developmental disabilities* [Paper presentation]. ObesityWeek 2018, Nashville, TN, United States.

Sherafat-Kazemzadeh, R., Yanovski, S. Z., & Yanovski, J. A. (2013). Pharmacotherapy for childhood obesity: Present and future prospects. *International Journal of Obesity, 37*(1), 1–15. https://doi.org/10.1038/ijo.2012.144

Sherar, L. B., Esliger, D. W., Baxter-Jones, A. D., & Tremblay, M. S. (2007). Age and gender differences in youth physical activity: Does physical maturity matter? *Medicine & Science in Sports & Exercise, 39*(5), 830–835. https://doi.org/10.1249/mss.0b013e3180335c3c

Shilts, M. K., Horowitz, M., & Townsend, M. S. (2004). Goal setting as a strategy for dietary and physical activity behavior change: A review of the literature. *American Journal of Health Promotion, 19*(2), 81–93. https://doi.org/10.4278/0890-1171-19.2.81

Shilts, M. K., Sitnic, S. L., Ontai, L., & Townsend, M. S. (2018). Guided goal setting: A feasible obesity prevention behavior change strategy for low-income parents with young children. *Journal of Human Sciences & Extension, 6*(3), 161–179. https://doi.org/10.54718/SKQL2392

Shomaker, L. B., Pivarunas, B., Annameier, S. K., Gulley, L., Quaglia, J., Brown, K. W., Broderick, P., & Bell, C. (2019). One-year follow-up of a randomized controlled trial piloting a mindfulness-based group intervention for adolescent insulin resistance. *Frontiers in Psychology, 10*, 1040. https://doi.org/10.3389/fpsyg.2019.01040

Showell, N. N., Fawole, O., Segal, J., Wilson, R. F., Cheskin, L. J., Bleich, S. N., Wu, Y., Lau, B., & Wang, Y. (2013). A systematic review of home-based childhood obesity prevention studies. *Pediatrics, 132*(1), e193–e200. https://doi.org/10.1542/peds.2013-0786

Sim, L. A., Lebow, J., & Billings, M. (2013). Eating disorders in adolescents with a history of obesity. *Pediatrics, 132*(4), e1026–e1030. https://doi.org/10.1542/peds.2012-3940

Singer, K., & Lumeng, C. N. (2017). The initiation of metabolic inflammation in childhood obesity. *The Journal of Clinical Investigation, 127*(1), 65–73. https://doi.org/10.1172/JCI88882

Singh, M. K., Leslie, S. M., Packer, M. M., Zaiko, Y. V., Phillips, O. R., Weisman, E. F., Wall, D. M., Jo, B., & Rasgon, N. (2019). Brain and behavioral correlates of insulin resistance in youth with depression and obesity. *Hormones and Behavior, 108*, 73–83. https://doi.org/10.1016/j.yhbeh.2018.03.009

Skeer, M. R., & Ballard, E. L. (2013). Are family meals as good for youth as we think they are? A review of the literature on family meals as they pertain to adolescent risk prevention. *Journal of Youth and Adolescence, 42*(7), 943–963. https://doi.org/10.1007/s10964-013-9963-z

Skinner, A. C., Perrin, E. M., Moss, L. A., & Skelton, J. A. (2015). Cardiometabolic risks and severity of obesity in children and young adults. *The New England Journal of Medicine, 373*(14), 1307–1317. https://doi.org/10.1056/NEJMoa1502821

Skinner, A. C., Ravanbakht, S. N., Skelton, J. A., Perrin, E. M., & Armstrong, S. C. (2018). Prevalence of obesity and severe obesity in US children, 1999–2016. *Pediatrics, 141*(3), e20173459. https://doi.org/10.1542/peds.2017-3459

Slaney, G., Salmon, J., & Weinstein, P. (2012). Can a school based programme in a natural environment reduce BMI in overweight adolescents? *Medical Hypotheses, 79*(1), 68–70. https://doi.org/10.1016/j.mehy.2012.04.002

Smink, F. R., van Hoeken, D., Oldehinkel, A. J., & Hoek, H. W. (2014). Prevalence and severity of *DSM-5* eating disorders in a community cohort of adolescents. *International Journal of Eating Disorders, 47*(6), 610–619. https://doi.org/10.1002/eat.22316

Smith, K. E., & Mason, T. B. (2022). Psychiatric comorbidity associated with weight status in 9 to 10 year old children. *Pediatric Obesity, 17*(5), 12883. https://doi.org/10.1111/ijpo.12883

Sonneville, K. R., Horton, N. J., Micali, N., Crosby, R. D., Swanson, S. A., Solmi, F., & Field, A. E. (2013). Longitudinal associations between binge eating and overeating and adverse outcomes among adolescents and young adults: Does loss of control matter? *JAMA Pediatrics, 167*(2), 149–155. https://doi.org/10.1001/2013.jamapediatrics.12

Sonneville, K. R., Thurston, I. B., Milliren, C. E., Kamody, R. C., Gooding, H. C., & Richmond, T. K. (2016). Helpful or harmful? Prospective association between weight misperception and weight gain among overweight and obese adolescents and young adults. *International Journal of Obesity, 40*(2), 328–332. https://doi.org/10.1038/ijo.2015.166

Spear, B. A., Barlow, S. E., Ervin, C., Ludwig, D. S., Saelens, B. E., Schetzina, K. E., & Taveras, E. M. (2007). Recommendations for treatment of child and adolescent overweight and obesity. *Pediatrics, 120*(Suppl. 4), S254–S288. https://doi.org/10.1542/peds.2007-2329F

Spitzer, R. L., Kroenke, K., Williams, J. B., & Löwe, B. (2006). A brief measure for assessing generalized anxiety disorder: The GAD-7. *Archives of Internal Medicine, 166*(10), 1092–1097. https://doi.org/10.1001/archinte.166.10.1092

Srivastava, G., Fox, C. K., Kelly, A. S., Jastreboff, A. M., Browne, A. F., Browne, N. T., Pratt, J. S. A., Bolling, C., Michalsky, M. P., Cook, S., Lenders, C. M., & Apovian, C. M. (2019). Clinical considerations regarding the use of obesity pharmacotherapy in adolescents with obesity. *Obesity, 27*(2), 190–204. https://doi.org/10.1002/oby.22385

Stark, L. J., Spear, S., Boles, R., Kuhl, E., Ratcliff, M., Scharf, C., Bolling, C., & Rausch, J. (2011). A pilot randomized controlled trial of a clinic and home-based behavioral intervention to decrease obesity in preschoolers. *Obesity, 19*(1), 134–141. https://doi.org/10.1038/oby.2010.87

Stice, E., Gau, J. M., Rohde, P., & Shaw, H. (2017). Risk factors that predict future onset of each *DSM-5* eating disorder: Predictive specificity in high-risk adolescent females. *Journal of Abnormal Psychology, 126*(1), 38–51. https://doi.org/10.1037/abn0000219

Stifter, C. A., Anzman-Frasca, S., Birch, L. L., & Voegtline, K. (2011). Parent use of food to soothe infant/toddler distress and child weight status. An exploratory study. *Appetite, 57*(3), 693–699. https://doi.org/10.1016/j.appet.2011.08.013

Strauss, W. J., Nagaraja, J., Landgraf, A. J., Arteaga, S. S., Fawcett, S. B., Ritchie, L. D., John, L. V., Gregoriou, M., Frongillo, E. A., Loria, C. M., Weber, S. A., Collie-Akers, V. L., McIver, K. L., Schultz, J., Sagatov, R. D. F., Leifer, E. S., Webb, K., Pate, R. R., & the Healthy Communities Study Team. (2018). The longitudinal relationship between community programmes and policies to prevent childhood obesity and BMI in children: The Healthy Communities Study. *Pediatric Obesity, 13*(Suppl. 1), 82–92. https://doi.org/10.1111/ijpo.12266

Styne, D. M., Arslanian, S. A., Connor, E. L., Farooqi, I. S., Murad, M. H., Silverstein, J. H., & Yanovski, J. A. (2017). Pediatric obesity—Assessment, treatment, and prevention: An Endocrine Society clinical practice guideline. *The Journal of Clinical Endocrinology & Metabolism, 102*(3), 709–757. https://doi.org/10.1210/jc.2016-2573

Su, S.-C., Sun, M.-T., Wen, M.-J., Lin, C.-J., Chen, Y.-C., & Hung, Y.-J. (2011). Brain-derived neurotrophic factor, adiponectin, and proinflammatory markers in various subtypes of depression in young men. *International Journal of Psychiatry in Medicine, 42*(3), 211–226. https://doi.org/10.2190/PM.42.3.a

Sun, A. P., Kirby, B., Black, C., Helms, P. J., Bennie, M., & McLay, J. S. (2014). Unplanned medication discontinuation as a potential pharmacovigilance signal: A nested young person cohort study. *BMC Pharmacology & Toxicology, 15*(1), 11. https://doi.org/10.1186/2050-6511-15-11

Swanson, S. A., Crow, S. J., Le Grange, D., Swendsen, J., & Merikangas, K. R. (2011). Prevalence and correlates of eating disorders in adolescents: Results from the National Comorbidity Survey Replication Adolescent Supplement. *Archives of General Psychiatry, 68*(7), 714–723. https://doi.org/10.1001/archgenpsychiatry.2011.22

Taddio, A., McMurtry, C. M., Logeman, C., Gudzak, V., de Boer, A., Constantin, K., Lee, S., Moline, R., Uleryk, E., Chera, T., MacDonald, N. E., & Pham, B. (2022). Prevalence of pain and fear as barriers to vaccination in children—Systematic review and meta-analysis. *Vaccine, 40*(52), 7526–7537. https://doi.org/10.1016/j.vaccine.2022.10.026

Taghizadeh, S., & Farhangi, M. A. (2020). The effectiveness of pediatric obesity prevention policies: A comprehensive systematic review and dose–response meta-analysis of controlled clinical trials. *Journal of Translational Medicine, 18*(1), 480. https://doi.org/10.1186/s12967-020-02640-1

Tanaka, V. T., Englehard, G., Jr., & Rabbitt, M. P. (2020). Using a bifactor model to measure food insecurity in households with children. *Journal of Family and Economic Issues, 41*(3), 492–504. https://doi.org/10.1007/s10834-020-09686-9

Tanas, R., Gil, B., Marsella, M., Nowicka, P., Pezzoli, V., Phelan, S. M., Queirolo, S., Stanford, F. C., Pettoello-Mantovani, M., & Bernasconi, S. (2022). Addressing weight stigma and weight-based discrimination in children: Preparing pediatricians to meet the challenge. *The Journal of Pediatrics, 248*, 135–136.e3. https://doi.org/10.1016/j.jpeds.2022.06.011

Taner, Y., Törel-Ergür, A., Bahçivan, G., & Gürdag, M. (2009). Psychopathology and its effect on treatment compliance in pediatric obesity patients. *The Turkish Journal of Pediatrics, 51*(5), 466–471.

Tanofsky-Kraff, M. (2008). Binge eating among children and adolescents. In *Handbook of childhood and adolescent obesity* (pp. 43–59). Springer. https://doi.org/10.1007/978-0-387-76924-0_4

Tanofsky-Kraff, M., Han, J. C., Anandalingam, K., Shomaker, L. B., Columbo, K. M., Wolkoff, L. E., Kozlosky, M., Elliott, C., Ranzenhofer, L. M., Roza, C. A., Yanovski, S. Z., & Yanovski, J. A. (2009). The FTO gene rs9939609 obesity-risk allele and loss of control over eating. *The American Journal of Clinical Nutrition, 90*(6), 1483–1488. https://doi.org/10.3945/ajcn.2009.28439

Tanofsky-Kraff, M., Shomaker, L. B., Wilfley, D. E., Young, J. F., Sbrocco, T., Stephens, M., Ranzenhofer, L. M., Elliott, C., Brady, S., Radin, R. M., Vannucci, A., Bryant, E. J., Osborn, R., Berger, S. S., Olsen, C., Kozlosky, M., Reynolds, J. C., & Yanovski, J. A. (2014). Targeted prevention of excess weight gain and eating disorders in high-risk adolescent girls: A randomized controlled trial. *The American Journal of Clinical Nutrition, 100*(4), 1010–1018. https://doi.org/10.3945/ajcn.114.092536

Taveras, E. M., Perkins, M. E., Boudreau, A. A., Blake-Lamb, T., Matathia, S., Kotelchuck, M., Luo, M., Price, S. N., Roche, B., & Cheng, E. R. (2021). Twelve-month outcomes of the First 1000 Days program on infant weight status. *Pediatrics, 148*(2), e2020046706. https://doi.org/10.1542/peds.2020-046706

Taylor, A., Wilson, C., Slater, A., & Mohr, P. (2012). Self-esteem and body dissatisfaction in young children: Associations with weight and perceived parenting style. *Clinical Psychologist, 16*(1), 25–35. https://doi.org/10.1111/j.1742-9552.2011.00038.x

Taylor, J. Y., Caldwell, C. H., Baser, R. E., Faison, N., & Jackson, J. S. (2007). Prevalence of eating disorders among Blacks in the National Survey of American Life. *International Journal of Eating Disorders, 40*(Suppl. 3), S10–S14. https://doi.org/10.1002/eat.20451

Taylor, N. J., Sahota, P., Sargent, J., Barber, S., Loach, J., Louch, G., & Wright, J. (2013). Using intervention mapping to develop a culturally appropriate intervention to prevent childhood obesity: The HAPPY (Healthy and Active Parenting Programme for Early Years) study. *International Journal of Behavioral Nutrition and Physical Activity, 10*(1), 1–16. https://doi.org/10.1186/1479-5868-10-142

Taylor, S. A., Ditch, S., & Hansen, S. (2018). Identifying and preventing eating disorders in adolescent patients with obesity. *Pediatric Annals, 47*(6), e232–e237. https://doi.org/10.3928/19382359-20180522-01

Terasaka, A., Tachibana, Y., Okuyama, M., & Igarashi, T. (2015). Post-traumatic stress disorder in children following natural disasters: A systematic review of the long-term follow-up studies. *International Journal of Child, Youth & Family Studies, 6*(1), 111–133. https://doi.org/10.18357/ijcyfs.61201513481

Tervalon, M., & Murray-García, J. (1998). Cultural humility versus cultural competence: A critical distinction in defining physician training outcomes in multicultural education. *Journal of Health Care for the Poor and Underserved, 9*(2), 117–125. https://doi.org/10.1353/hpu.2010.0233

Thaker, V. V. (2017). Genetic and epigenetic causes of obesity. *Adolescent Medicine: State of the Art Reviews, 28*(2), 379–405. https://www.ncbi.nlm.nih.gov/pubmed/30416642

Thomas, C. E., Mauer, E. A., Shukla, A. P., Rathi, S., & Aronne, L. J. (2016). Low adoption of weight loss medications: A comparison of prescribing patterns of antiobesity pharmacotherapies and SGLT2s. *Obesity, 24*(9), 1955–1961. https://doi.org/10.1002/oby.21533

Thomas, E. E., Haydon, H. M., Mehrotra, A., Caffery, L. J., Snoswell, C. L., Banbury, A., & Smith, A. C. (2022). Building on the momentum: Sustaining telehealth beyond COVID-19. *Journal of Telemedicine and Telecare, 28*(4), 301–308. https://doi.org/10.1177/1357633X20960638

Thompson, I., Hong, J. S., Lee, J. M., Prys, N. A., Morgan, J. T., & Udo-Inyang, I. (2020). A review of the empirical research on weight-based bullying and peer victimisation published between 2006 and 2016. *Educational Review, 72*(1), 88–110. https://doi.org/10.1080/00131911.2018.1483894

Thompson, S. H., Corwin, S. J., & Sargent, R. G. (1997). Ideal body size beliefs and weight concerns of fourth-grade children. *International Journal of Eating Disorders, 21*(3), 279–284. https://doi.org/10.1002/(SICI)1098-108X(199704)21:3<279::AID-EAT8>3.0.CO;2-H

Thurston, I. B., Sonneville, K. R., Milliren, C. E., Kamody, R. C., Gooding, H. C., & Richmond, T. K. (2017). Cross-sectional and prospective examination of weight misperception and depressive symptoms among youth with overweight and obesity. *Prevention Science, 18*(2), 152–163. https://doi.org/10.1007/s11121-016-0714-8

Tomiyama, A. J., Carr, D., Granberg, E. M., Major, B., Robinson, E., Sutin, A. R., & Brewis, A. (2018). How and why weight stigma drives the obesity "epidemic" and harms health. *BMC Medicine, 16*(1), 123. https://doi.org/10.1186/s12916-018-1116-5

Torbic, H. (2011). Children and grief: But what about the children? *Home Healthcare Now, 29*(2), 67–77. https://doi.org/10.1097/NHH.0b013e31820861dd

Tork, S., Meister, K. M., Uebele, A. L., Hussain, L. R., Kelley, S. R., Kerlakian, G. M., & Tymitz, K. M. (2015). Factors influencing primary care physicians' referral for bariatric surgery. *Journal of the Society of Laparoendoscopic Surgeons, 19*(3), e2015.00046. https://doi.org/10.4293/JSLS.2015.00046

Trace, S. E., Thornton, L. M., Root, T. L., Mazzeo, S. E., Lichtenstein, P., Pedersen, N. L., & Bulik, C. M. (2012). Effects of reducing the frequency and duration criteria for binge eating on lifetime prevalence of bulimia nervosa and binge eating disorder: Implications for *DSM-5*. *International Journal of Eating Disorders, 45*(4), 531–536. https://doi.org/10.1002/eat.20955

Trasande, L., & Chatterjee, S. (2009). The impact of obesity on health service utilization and costs in childhood. *Obesity, 17*(9), 1749–1754. https://doi.org/10.1038/oby.2009.67

Tronieri, J., Wadden, T., Leonard, S., & Berkowitz, R. (2019). A pilot study of acceptance-based behavioural weight loss for adolescents with obesity. *Behavioural and Cognitive Psychotherapy, 47*(6), 686–696. https://doi.org/10.1017/S1352465819000262

Trost, S. G., Sallis, J. F., Pate, R. R., Freedson, P. S., Taylor, W. C., & Dowda, M. (2003). Evaluating a model of parental influence on youth physical activity. *American Journal of Preventive Medicine, 25*(4), 277–282. https://doi.org/10.1016/s0749-3797(03)00217-4

Tucker, J. M., Stratbucker, W., King, E. C., Cuda, S., Negrete, S., Sweeney, B., Kumar, S., Borzutzky, C., Binns, H. J., Kirk, S., & the POWER Work Group. (2022). Characteristics of paediatric weight management in the United States: Associations with program retention and BMI outcomes in the Paediatric Obesity Weight Evaluation Registry (POWER). *Pediatric Obesity, 17*(2), e12848. https://doi.org/10.1111/ijpo.12848

Tulving, E. (2002). Episodic memory: From mind to brain. *Annual Review of Psychology, 53*(1), 1–25. https://doi.org/10.1146/annurev.psych.53.100901.135114

Turner, T., Spruijt-Metz, D., Wen, C. K., & Hingle, M. D. (2015). Prevention and treatment of pediatric obesity using mobile and wireless technologies: A systematic review. *Pediatric Obesity, 10*(6), 403–409. https://doi.org/10.1111/ijpo.12002

Tutlam, N. T., Liu, Y., Nelson, E. J., Flick, L. H., & Chang, J. J. (2017). The effects of race and ethnicity on the risk of large-for-gestational-age newborns in women without gestational diabetes by prepregnancy body mass index categories. *Maternal and Child Health Journal, 21*(8), 1643–1654. https://doi.org/10.1007/s10995-016-2256-x

U.S. Centers for Disease Control and Prevention. (2012). File: Medical complications of obesity.png. In *Wikimedia Commons*. https://commons.wikimedia.org/wiki/File:Medical_complications_of_obesity.png

U.S. Centers for Disease Control and Prevention. (2017). *Picture of America: Prevention*. https://www.cdc.gov/pictureofamerica/pdfs/picture_of_america_prevention.pdf

U.S. Centers for Disease Control and Prevention. (2021). *Whole school, whole community, whole child (WSCC)*. https://www.cdc.gov/healthyschools/wscc/index.htm

U.S. Centers for Disease Control and Prevention. (2022a). *Fast facts: Preventing adverse childhood experiences*. https://www.cdc.gov/violenceprevention/aces/fastfact.html

U.S. Centers for Disease Control and Prevention. (2022b). *What is health equity?* https://www.cdc.gov/healthequity/whatis/index.html

U.S. Centers for Disease Control and Prevention. (2022c). *Your baby at 2 months.* https://www.cdc.gov/ncbddd/actearly/pdf/FULL-LIST-CDC_LTSAE-Checklists2021_Eng_FNL2_508.pdf

U.S. Centers for Medicare & Medicaid Services. (2023). *Reducing obesity.* https://www.medicaid.gov/medicaid/quality-of-care/quality-improvement-initiatives/reducing-obesity/index.html

van Dijk, S. J., Molloy, P. L., Varinli, H., Morrison, J. L., Muhlhausler, B. S., Buckley, M., Clark, S. J., McMillen, I. C., Noakes, M., Samaras, K., Tellam, R. L., & the Members of EpiSCOPE. (2015). Epigenetics and human obesity. *International Journal of Obesity, 39*(1), 85–97. https://doi.org/10.1038/ijo.2014.34

Vartanian, L. R., Pinkus, R. T., & Smyth, J. M. (2014). The phenomenology of weight stigma in everyday life. *Journal of Contextual Behavioral Science, 3*(3), 196–202. https://doi.org/10.1016/j.jcbs.2014.01.003

Vazquez, C. E., & Cubbin, C. (2020). Socioeconomic status and childhood obesity: A review of literature from the past decade to inform intervention research. *Current Obesity Reports, 9*(4), 562–570. https://doi.org/10.1007/s13679-020-00400-2

Venturelli, F., Ferrari, F., Broccoli, S., Bonvicini, L., Mancuso, P., Bargellini, A., & Giorgi Rossi, P. (2019). The effect of public health/pediatric obesity interventions on socioeconomic inequalities in childhood obesity: A scoping review. *Obesity Reviews, 20*(12), 1720–1739. https://doi.org/10.1111/obr.12931

Verbiest, I., Michels, N., Tanghe, A., & Braet, C. (2021). Inflammation in obese children and adolescents: Association with psychosocial stress variables and effects of a lifestyle intervention. *Brain, Behavior, and Immunity, 98*, 40–47. https://doi.org/10.1016/j.bbi.2021.07.020

Viswanathan, S., McNelis, K., Makker, K., Calhoun, D., Woo, J. G., & Balagopal, B. (2022). Childhood obesity and adverse cardiometabolic risk in large for gestational age infants and potential early preventive strategies: A narrative review. *Pediatric Research, 92*(3), 653–661. https://doi.org/10.1038/s41390-021-01904-w

Vogel, E. N., Singh, S., & Accurso, E. C. (2021). A systematic review of cognitive behavior therapy and dialectical behavior therapy for adolescent eating disorders. *Journal of Eating Disorders, 9*(1), 131. https://doi.org/10.1186/s40337-021-00461-1

Vuong, L., Chang, S. H., Wan, F., Wu, N., Eagon, J. C., Eckhouse, S. R., & Dimou, F. M. (2022). National trends and outcomes in adolescents undergoing bariatric surgery. *Journal of the American College of Surgeons, 235*(2), 186–194. https://doi.org/10.1097/XCS.0000000000000234

Wade, C., Burton, E. T., Akinseye, L., Nelson, G., Smith-Young, J., & Kim, A. (2022). Increased anxiety symptoms in pediatric type 1 diabetes during the acute phase of COVID-19 lockdown. *Journal of Pediatric Endocrinology & Metabolism, 35*(5), 627–630. https://doi.org/10.1515/jpem-2022-0002

Walker, L. L., Gately, P. J., Bewick, B. M., & Hill, A. J. (2003). Children's weight-loss camps: Psychological benefit or jeopardy? *International Journal of Obesity, 27*(6), 748–754. https://doi.org/10.1038/sj.ijo.0802290

Walsh, R. (2011). Lifestyle and mental health. *American Psychologist, 66*(7), 579–592. https://doi.org/10.1037/a0021769

Wang, F., & Veugelers, P. J. (2008). Self-esteem and cognitive development in the era of the childhood obesity epidemic. *Obesity Reviews, 9*(6), 615–623. https://doi.org/10.1111/j.1467-789X.2008.00507.x

Wang, H., Guo, J., Guo, Y., Lv, W., Jiang, Y., & Whittemore, R. (2021). Effectiveness of family systems theory interventions on adolescents with type 1 diabetes: A meta-analysis. *Journal of Child and Family Studies, 30*(11), 2664–2676. https://doi.org/10.1007/s10826-021-02069-0

Wang, X., Cai, Z. D., Jiang, W. T., Fang, Y. Y., Sun, W. X., & Wang, X. (2022). Systematic review and meta-analysis of the effects of exercise on depression in adolescents. *Child and Adolescent Psychiatry and Mental Health, 16*(1), 16. https://doi.org/10.1186/s13034-022-00453-2

Wang, Y., Beydoun, M. A., Liang, L., Caballero, B., & Kumanyika, S. K. (2008). Will all Americans become overweight or obese? Estimating the progression and cost of the US obesity epidemic. *Obesity, 16*(10), 2323–2330. https://doi.org/10.1038/oby.2008.351

Wang, Y., Cai, L., Wu, Y., Wilson, R. F., Weston, C., Fawole, O., Bleich, S. N., Cheskin, L. J., Showell, N. N., Lau, B. D., Chiu, D. T., Zhang, A., & Segal, J. (2015). What childhood obesity prevention programmes work? A systematic review and meta-analysis. *Obesity Reviews, 16*(7), 547–565. https://doi.org/10.1111/obr.12277

Ward, Z. J., Rodriguez, P., Wright, D. R., Austin, S. B., & Long, M. W. (2019). Estimation of eating disorders prevalence by age and associations with mortality in a simulated nationally representative US cohort. *JAMA Network Open, 2*(10), e1912925. https://doi.org/10.1001/jamanetworkopen.2019.12925

Wardle, J., Guthrie, C. A., Sanderson, S., & Rapoport, L. (2001). Development of the Children's Eating Behaviour Questionnaire. *Journal of Child Psychology and Psychiatry, 42*(7), 963–970. https://doi.org/10.1111/1469-7610.00792

Warnick, J. L., Darling, K. E., West, C. E., Jones, L., & Jelalian, E. (2022). Weight stigma and mental health in youth: A systematic review and meta-analysis. *Journal of Pediatric Psychology, 47*(3), 237–255. https://doi.org/10.1093/jpepsy/jsab110

Webb, K. L., Hewawitharana, S. C., Au, L. E., Collie-Akers, V., Strauss, W. J., Landgraf, A. J., Nagaraja, J., Wilson, D. K., Sagatov, R., Kao, J., Loria, C. M., Fawcett, S. B., Ritchie, L. D., & the Healthy Communities Study Team. (2018). Objectives of community policies and programs associated with more healthful dietary intakes among children: Findings from the Healthy Communities Study. *Pediatric Obesity, 13*(Suppl. 1), 103–112. https://doi.org/10.1111/ijpo.12424

Weghuber, D., Barrett, T., Barrientos-Pérez, M., Gies, I., Hesse, D., Jeppesen, O. K., Kelly, A. S., Mastrandrea, L. D., Sørrig, R., Arslanian, S., & the STEP TEENS Investigators. (2022). Once-weekly semaglutide in adolescents with obesity. *The New England Journal of Medicine, 387*(24), 2245–2257. https://doi.org/10.1056/NEJMoa2208601

Wehrly, S. E., Bonilla, C., Perez, M., & Liew, J. (2014). Controlling parental feeding practices and child body composition in ethnically and economically diverse preschool children. *Appetite, 73*, 163–171. https://doi.org/10.1016/j.appet.2013.11.009

White, G. E., Boles, R. E., Courcoulas, A. P., Yanovski, S. Z., Zeller, M. H., Jenkins, T. M., & Inge, T. H. (2023). A Prospective Cohort of Alcohol use and Alcohol-related Problems Before and After Metabolic and Bariatric Surgery in Adolescents. *Annals of Surgery, 278*(3), e519–e525. https://doi.org/10.1097/SLA.0000000000005759

Whitlock, E. P., O'Connor, E. A., Williams, S. B., Beil, T. L., & Lutz, K. W. (2010). Effectiveness of weight management interventions in children: A targeted systematic review for the USPSTF. *Pediatrics, 125*(2), e396–e418. https://doi.org/10.1542/peds.2009-1955

Wilding, J. P. H., Batterham, R. L., Davies, M., Van Gaal, L. F., Kandler, K., Konakli, K., Lingvay, I., McGowan, B. M., Oral, T. K., Rosenstock, J., Wadden, T. A., Wharton, S., Yokote, K., Kushner, R. F., & the STEP 1 Study Group. (2022). Weight regain and cardiometabolic effects after withdrawal of semaglutide: The STEP 1 trial extension. *Diabetes, Obesity & Metabolism, 24*(8), 1553–1564. https://doi.org/10.1111/dom.14725

Wilfley, D. E., Citrome, L., & Herman, B. K. (2016). Characteristics of binge eating disorder in relation to diagnostic criteria. *Neuropsychiatric Disease and Treatment, 12*, 2213–2223. https://doi.org/10.2147/NDT.S107777

Williams-Kerver, G. A., Steffen, K. J., & Mitchell, J. E. (2019). Eating pathology after bariatric surgery: An updated review of the recent literature. *Current Psychiatry Reports, 21*(9), 86. https://doi.org/10.1007/s11920-019-1071-7

Wilson, D. K., & Lawman, H. G. (2009). Health promotion in children and adolescents: An integration of the biopsychosocial model and ecological approaches to behavior change. In M. C. Roberts & R. G. Steele (Eds.), *Handbook of pediatric psychology* (4th ed., pp. 603–617). Guilford Press.

Wingrave, P. (2023, June 27). Focus: Obesity drug Wegovy's popularity has US employers rethinking insurance coverage. Reuters. https://www.reuters.com/business/healthcare-pharmaceuticals/obesity-drug-wegovys-popularity-has-us-employers-rethinking-insurance-coverage-2023-06-27/

Wolch, J., Jerrett, M., Reynolds, K., McConnell, R., Chang, R., Dahmann, N., Brady, K., Gilliland, F., Su, J. G., & Berhane, K. (2011). Childhood obesity and proximity to urban parks and recreational resources: A longitudinal cohort study. *Health & Place, 17*(1), 207–214. https://doi.org/10.1016/j.healthplace.2010.10.001

Wolkoff, L. E., Tanofsky-Kraff, M., Shomaker, L. B., Kozlosky, M., Columbo, K. M., Elliott, C. A., Ranzenhofer, L. M., Osborn, R. L., Yanovski, S. Z., & Yanovski, J. A. (2011). Self-reported vs. actual energy intake in youth with and without loss of control eating. *Eating Behaviors, 12*(1), 15–20. https://doi.org/10.1016/j.eatbeh.2010.09.001

Wolraich, M. L., Lambert, W., Doffing, M. A., Bickman, L., Simmons, T., & Worley, K. (2003). Psychometric properties of the Vanderbilt ADHD diagnostic parent rating scale in a referred population. *Journal of Pediatric Psychology, 28*(8), 559–568. https://doi.org/10.1093/jpepsy/jsg046

Wood, A. C., Vainik, U., Engelhardt, L. E., Briley, D. A., Grotzinger, A. D., Church, J. A., Harden, K. P., & Tucker-Drob, E. M. (2019). Genetic overlap between executive functions and BMI in childhood. *The American Journal of Clinical Nutrition, 110*(4), 814–822. https://doi.org/10.1093/ajcn/nqz109

Woolford, S. J., Clark, S. J., Gebremariam, A., Davis, M. M., & Freed, G. L. (2010). To cut or not to cut: Physicians' perspectives on referring adolescents for bariatric surgery. *Obesity Surgery, 20*(7), 937–942. https://doi.org/10.1007/s11695-010-0152-9

Woolford, S. J., Clark, S. J., Sallinen, B. J., Geiger, J. D., & Freed, G. L. (2012). Bariatric surgery decision making challenges: The stability of teens' decisions and the treatment failure paradox. *Pediatric Surgery International, 28*(5), 455–460. https://doi.org/10.1007/s00383-012-3069-7

World Cancer Research Fund International. (2022). *MOVING Framework.* https://www.wcrf.org/policy/policy-databases/moving-framework/

World Health Organization. (2021, June 9). *Obesity and overweight.* https://www.who.int/news-room/fact-sheets/detail/obesity-and-overweight

World Health Organization Commission on Ending Childhood Obesity. (2017). *Report of the commission on ending childhood obesity.* https://apps.who.int/iris/bitstream/10665/204176/1/9789241510066_eng.pdf?ua=1

World Health Organization Regional Office for Europe. (2017). *Weight bias and obesity stigma: Considerations for the WHO European Region.* https://iris.who.int/bitstream/handle/10665/353613/WHO-EURO-2022-5369-45134-64401-eng.pdf?sequence=1

Wright, D. R., Guo, J., & Hernandez, I. (2023). A prescription for achieving equitable access to antiobesity medications. *JAMA Health Forum, 4*(4), e230493. https://doi.org/10.1001/jamahealthforum.2023.0493

Wu, X., Bastian, K., Ohinmaa, A., & Veugelers, P. (2018). Influence of physical activity, sedentary behavior, and diet quality in childhood on the incidence of internalizing and externalizing disorders during adolescence: A population-based cohort study. *Annals of Epidemiology, 28*(2), 86–94. https://doi.org/10.1016/j.annepidem.2017.12.002

Wu, Y., Perng, W., & Peterson, K. E. (2020). Precision nutrition and childhood obesity: A scoping review. *Metabolites, 10*(6), 235. https://doi.org/10.3390/metabo10060235

Xanthakos, S. A., Khoury, J. C., Inge, T. H., Jenkins, T. M., Modi, A. C., Michalsky, M. P., Chen, M. K., Courcoulas, A. P., Harmon, C. M., & Brandt, M. L. (2020). Nutritional risks in adolescents after bariatric surgery. *Clinical Gastroenterology and Hepatology, 18*(5), 1070–1081. https://doi.org/10.1016/j.cgh.2019.10.048

Xin, J., Zhao, L., Wu, T., Zhang, L., Li, Y., Xue, H., Xiao, Q., Wang, R., Xu, P., Visscher, T., Ma, X., & Jia, P. (2021). Association between access to convenience stores and childhood obesity: A systematic review. *Obesity Reviews, 22*(Suppl. 1), e12908. https://doi.org/10.1111/obr.12908

Yanovski, S. Z., Marcus, M. D., Wadden, T. A., & Walsh, B. T. (2015). The Questionnaire on Eating and Weight Patterns-5: An updated screening instrument for binge eating disorder. *International Journal of Eating Disorders, 48*(3), 259–261. https://doi.org/10.1002/eat.22372

Yearby, R. (2018). Racial disparities in health status and access to healthcare: The continuation of inequality in the United States due to structural racism. *American Journal of Economics and Sociology, 77*(3–4), 1113–1152. https://doi.org/10.1111/ajes.12230

Yi, D. Y., Kim, S. C., Lee, J. H., Lee, E. H., Kim, J. Y., Kim, Y. J., Kang, K. S., Hong, J., Shim, J. O., Lee, Y., Kang, B., Lee, Y. J., Kim, M. J., Moon, J. S., Koh, H., You, J., Kwak, Y. S., Lim, H., & Yang, H. R. (2019). Clinical practice guideline for the diagnosis and treatment of pediatric obesity: Recommendations from the Committee on Pediatric Obesity of the Korean Society of Pediatric Gastroenterology Hepatology and Nutrition. *Korean Journal of Pediatrics, 62*(1), 3–21. https://doi.org/10.3345/kjp.2018.07360

Zavodny, M. (2013). Does weight affect children's test scores and teacher assessments differently? *Economics of Education Review, 34*, 135–145. https://doi.org/10.1016/j.econedurev.2013.02.003

Zeller, M. H., Brown, J. L., Reiter-Purtill, J., Sarwer, D. B., Black, L., Jenkins, T. M., McCracken, K. A., Courcoulas, A. P., Inge, T. H., Noll, J. G., Doland, F., Morgenthal, A., Howarth, T., Comstock, S., Kirk, S., Helmrath, M., Lee, M. C., Allen, D., Garland, B., . . . Akers, R. (2019). Sexual behaviors, risks, and sexual health outcomes for adolescent females following bariatric surgery. *Surgery for Obesity and Related Diseases, 15*(6), 969–978. https://doi.org/10.1016/j.soard.2019.03.001

Zeller, M. H., Reiter-Purtill, J., Jenkins, T. M., Kidwell, K. M., Bensman, H. E., Mitchell, J. E., Courcoulas, A. P., Inge, T. H., Ley, S. L., Gordon, K. H., Chaves, E. A., Washington, G. A., Austin, H. M., & Rofey, D. L. (2020). Suicidal thoughts and behaviors in adolescents who underwent bariatric surgery. *Surgery for Obesity and Related Diseases, 16*(4), 568–580. https://doi.org/10.1016/j.soard.2019.12.015

Zeller, M. H., Reiter-Purtill, J., Jenkins, T. M., & Ratcliff, M. B. (2013). Adolescent suicidal behavior across the excess weight status spectrum. *Obesity, 21*(5), 1039–1045. https://doi.org/10.1002/oby.20084

Zeller, M. H., Roehrig, H. R., Modi, A. C., Daniels, S. R., & Inge, T. H. (2006). Health-related quality of life and depressive symptoms in adolescents with extreme obesity presenting for bariatric surgery. *Pediatrics, 117*(4), 1155–1161. https://doi.org/10.1542/peds.2005-1141

Zhao, X., Page, T. F., Altszuler, A. R., Pelham, W. E., III, Kipp, H., Gnagy, E. M., Coxe, S., Schatz, N. K., Merrill, B. M., Macphee, F. L., & Pelham, W. E., Jr. (2019). Family burden of raising a child with ADHD. *Journal of Abnormal Child Psychology, 47*(8), 1327–1338. https://doi.org/10.1007/s10802-019-00518-5

Zhou, Y. E., Emerson, J. S., Levine, R. S., Kihlberg, C. J., & Hull, P. C. (2014). Childhood obesity prevention interventions in childcare settings: Systematic review of randomized and nonrandomized controlled trials. *American Journal of Health Promotion, 28*(4), e92–e103. https://doi.org/10.4278/ajhp.121129-LIT-579

Zickgraf, H., & Mayes, S. D. (2019). Psychological, health, and demographic correlates of atypical eating behaviors in children with autism. *Journal of Developmental and Physical Disabilities, 31*(3), 399–418. https://doi.org/10.1007/s10882-018-9645-6

Zoogman, S., Goldberg, S. B., Hoyt, W. T., & Miller, L. (2015). Mindfulness interventions with youth: A meta-analysis. *Mindfulness, 6*(2), 290–302. https://doi.org/10.1007/s12671-013-0260-4

Zubler, J. M., Wiggins, L. D., Macias, M. M., Whitaker, T. M., Shaw, J. S., Squires, J. K., Pajek, J. A., Wolf, R. B., Slaughter, K. S., Broughton, A. S., Gerndt, K. L., Mlodoch, B. J., & Lipkin, P. H. (2022). Evidence-informed milestones for developmental surveillance tools. *Pediatrics, 149*(3), e2021052138. https://doi.org/10.1542/peds.2021-052138

Index

A

About the Authors

Dr. Crystal S. Lim is chair and associate professor in the Department of Health Psychology in the College of Health Sciences at the University of Missouri. She has been working with children with overweight and obesity and their caregivers for more than 15 years in community-based and clinical settings. Dr. Lim is a licensed psychologist and is board certified in clinical child and adolescent psychology. She provides psychological services focused on weight management to youth and families. Dr. Lim is the director of the Mizzou Health Psychology Research Lab and conducts research that examines medical and psychological comorbidities in pediatric obesity, and she develops, implements, and evaluates family-based weight management interventions. Dr. Lim is actively involved in training undergraduate and graduate students, psychology interns, and postdoctoral fellows in clinical service, research, and professional development. Dr. Lim received her PhD in clinical psychology from Georgia State University and completed postdoctoral training in pediatric psychology at the University of Florida.

Dr. E. Thomaseo Burton is an assistant professor in the Department of Child and Adolescent Psychiatry and Behavioral Sciences, Perelman School of Medicine, at the University of Pennsylvania. Trained as a clinical psychologist, Dr. Burton's research seeks to develop and implement high-quality and culturally relevant behavioral interventions for children, adolescents, and their families with overweight, obesity, and related cardiometabolic comorbidities; he has a particular interest in mindfulness-based interventions. Dr. Burton serves as pediatric psychologist for the Healthy Weight Program at Children's Hospital of Philadelphia. He is committed to increasing representation of psychologists of color and actively mentors and supervises psychology trainees, from high school to postdoctoral fellowship. Dr. Burton earned a PhD in clinical psychology from Purdue University as well as master of public health degree with a focus on community health. He completed postdoctoral training in pediatric obesity at Boston Children's Hospital/ Harvard Medical School. Dr. Burton is board certified in Clinical Child and Adolescent Psychology by the American Board of Professional Psychology.